UNEMPLOYMENT AND HEALTH

A Disaster and a Challenge

RICHARD SMITH

Assistant editor, British Medical Journal

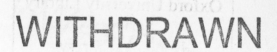

Oxford New York Tokyo
OXFORD UNIVERSITY PRESS
1987

Oxford University Press, Walton Street, Oxford OX2 6DP

Oxford New York Toronto
Delhi Bombay Calcutta Madras Karachi
Petaling Jaya Singapore Hong Kong Tokyo
Nairobi Dar es Salaam Cape Town
Melbourne Auckland

and associated companies in
Beirut Berlin Ibadan Nicosia

Oxford is a trade mark of Oxford University Press

British Library Cataloguing in Publication Data
Smith, Richard, 1952-
Unemployment and health, a disaster and a challenge.—
(Oxford medical publications).
1. Unemployed—Health and hygiene
i. Title
613   RC963.6.U5
ISBN 0-19-261622-6

Typeset by Downdell Ltd. Abingdon Oxon.
Printed in Great Britain by
Richard Clay Ltd.
Bungay, Suffolk.

Foreword

DEREK WORLOCK
Archbishop of Liverpool

DAVID SHEPPARD
Bishop of Liverpool

THE steady rise in long-term unemployment in recent years has led to many attempts to gauge the effect of joblessness on the attitude and habits of the unemployed. Some of these have been concerned with the psychological effects, others with the effects on human relationships, especially within family life. The resulting assessments have not been unanimous. Often there is something of the 'chicken and the egg' in the uncertainty as to which causes what. General agreement seems confined to the firm if simple belief that, in accord with the individual's circumstances and environment, being without a job operates to a person's disadvantage. This is expressed most commonly by the assertion that over a long time the unemployed person is in danger of losing the desire and to some extent the capacity for work. But even this generalization is challenged by the fact that an advertisement of a worthwhile job is frequently over applied for by ordinary and semiskilled or unskilled workers.

All manner of human reasons can be advanced as to why an unemployed person becomes discouraged after making a number of unsuccessful applications for a job. But it seems sadly true that when hope and the spirit of initiative are crushed, the jobless can all too easily pass from the status of unemployed to that of unemployable. The effect on the family of the father's being unable to secure work over a long period takes a predictable pattern. Father John Fitzsimons, a well-known priest–sociologist in Liverpool, has written: 'The psychology of the individual who finds his job disappear is fairly well established. At first, for some three months or so, he feels that the situation is transitory and he is kept going by energetic hope. The next six to nine months bring increasing despair, and after a year or so gives way to lethargy and a feeling of rejection.'[1]

The same report indicates evidence of the strain on marriage of the unemployment of middle-aged men. The relationship of a couple has usually been built upon a certain pattern where the man is the main bread-winner. For the greater part of the day he is away from home and is not in for his midday meal. If he becomes unemployed he is home nearly all the time and new adjustments have to be made. The man may feel rejected by his wife in addition to his rejection by society. The unease, short temper, dejectedness, and frustration overflow into relations with the children. If they are young, they are pushed on to the streets for longer periods; if they are adolescent, there will often be confrontations, verbal and at times even violent. Where there has been no true partnership with the wife, husbands can develop a sense of guilt which leads to estrangement.

It is inevitable that strain of this kind should have some effect upon health. But what precisely? In this series of articles, now brought together as a book, Dr Richard Smith endeavours to take the study a stage further. He asks whether unemployment is more an economic than a medical problem and tells of the undoubted association of unemployment with ill health. To some extent he too moves towards 'the chicken and the egg' problem, recognizing that ill health can be the cause of unemployment as well as being the result of it.

The overall impression of these papers is that the whole complex problem of unemployment is often the occasion of mental and physical illness, if not actually the obvious cause of it. Many social factors conspire to bring about ill health and the effects of being unemployed cannot be separated from the effects of poverty, poor housing, environment, poor nutrition, etc. We have already quoted Father Fitzsimons on the psychological processes that follow unemployment. Dr Smith explores this same cyclic problem where a job can cause stress, stress can lead to ill health and loss of job, which in turn add up to further illness which gives way to an attitude of seemingly being unemployable. But even the extensive use of researched statistics, for example, the comparative figures of sickness amongst employed and unemployed, does not produce conclusive evidence.

Some important points, however, are made in the course of this study, and none more important than the fact that in considering statistics we are talking of people. The author points out that it is the health of the whole person which is at stake; that the worry in advance about possible redundancy is often more damaging to health than is unemployment itself. Also (in our experience this is quite common), he points out that unemployment can hit at a man's dignity and self-esteem, and being without occupation can lead to a sense of being unwanted and a lack of fulfilment.

An interesting distinction is made between the effect of long-term unemployment and the effects associated with being between jobs for a short period. Prolonged unemployment can produce the kind of apathy and 'aggressive' self-defence that destroys family harmony. The shorter term between-jobs situation can give rise to uncertainty and even acute anxiety. The interplay of physical and mental effects is obvious. The author of these studies, in surveying the evidence, tries to avoid easy generalizations but establishes the undoubted relationship between ill health and unemployment.

Professor Alwyn Smith, in introducing the work of the Unemployment and Health Study Group, makes the point that unemployment on the present scale implies not simply an unequal distribution of work but, more significantly, inequalities both in income and in health.[2] To take steps to reduce the effects of unemployment is to safeguard the health of the workforce of the nation. If, as is our belief, there is no foreseeable return to full employment of the conventional kind, politicians, economists, and social workers will have to work alongside medicine—and, dare we say, the Church—to reduce the misery of unemployment and find alternatives to traditional employment.

References

1. Merseyside Enterprise Forum. *Chips with everything: a report on the social implications of advancing technology.* Liverpool: Merseyside Enterprise Forum, 1980.

2. Unemployment and Health Study Group. *Unemployment, health, and social policy.* Leeds: Nuffield Centre for Health Service Studies, 1984.

Contents

1

Bitterness, shame, emptiness, waste
An introduction to unemployment
and health

EMPLOYMENT matters to the individual more than government, education, religion, defence, and even health. It is, as the distinguished sociologist Marie Jahoda has said, 'the central institution' in industrial societies. We define ourselves through our employment. The first question asked of a stranger is usually, 'What do you do?' And the person asked the question understands that he is being asked about his employment, not about anything else he might do, think, or believe. Purpose, status, income, social contact, a structure to our days and lives, and a sense of belonging all come primarily from employment. Our education is understood to be preparing us for employment, and a pension comes once we have completed our allotted span of employment. The time of the community as well as the time of the individual is organized around employment: the crucial division is between 'the working week' and the weekend; Christmas for most people has more to do with 'time off' than religion; and—until very recently—television began once the working day was over. Employment might even be called the glue that keeps our society together.

Once it is understood that employment has been the most important institution in industrialized countries for more than a century, it is easy to see why the unemployed—those who are shut out—are so miserable. Being unemployed may be worse than being excommunicated, disenfranchized, illiterate, conquered, and even diseased. You do not belong and you are not wanted. Many unemployed people feel that their lives have neither structure nor purpose. It is a matter of dragging through a lifetime of impoverished days. To 'live again' you must get a job or start to think completely afresh.

This understanding of the importance of employment is the most significant insight that I have gained from researching this book, which has grown from 14 articles originally published in the *British Medical Journal*. Like many insights that are hard won it now seems almost obvious, but it has taken me many months of conversation, interviews, and reading to reach. A quicker way to reach the same conclusion is to lose your job and spend months unemployed—in the same way that people first understand the importance of health or a relationship when they lose one or the other. But, despite more than three million people being unemployed in Britain, most people (and probably most readers of this book) have not spent long spells unemployed. This is particularly true of health workers, who will, I hope, make up one of the main audiences of this book. It is also true of many of the country's 'decision-makers'. Many people have thus not understood the centrality of employment. Many persist, too, in feeling hostile towards the unemployed, being convinced that they are 'scroungers', that 'it's their own fault', and 'they could get a job if they really wanted one'.

A danger we must all avoid with the present concentration on unemployment is to glorify and romanticize employment. Most employment for most people has since the industrial revolution been hard, exhausting, boring, dirty, degrading, and, as Marx said, alienating. William Faulkner wrote: 'You can't eat for eight hours a day nor make love for eight hours a day—all you can do for eight hours is work. Which is the reason why man makes himself and everybody else so miserable and unhappy.'

Voltaire, Carlyle, and Tolstoy all took a very different view. Voltaire wrote that 'work banishes those three great evils, boredom, vice, and poverty', while Carlyle claimed that 'work is the grand cure of all the maladies and miseries that ever beset mankind'. Tolstoy in *War and Peace* has Prince Andrei's father say: 'Only fools and rakes ever need be ill, my boy, and you know me—abstemious, and busy from morning till night, so of course I'm well.'

Another great writer, Albert Camus, explains these contradictions by what he says about work: 'Without work all life goes rotten, but when work is soulless, life stifles and dies.' The work that Voltaire, Carlyle, and Tolstoy enjoyed was very different from that of a Victorian child up a chimney or a convict breaking up rocks.

We must be careful of this word 'work', which brings me to a second important insight that I have gained, which again now seems obvious. It is that employment and work are not the same. As the late Sir Desmond Pond, former chief scientist and president of the Royal College of Psychiatrists, put it: 'There are many employed people who do not work and many unemployed people who work round the clock—perhaps looking after their children or a sick relative.' Yet if you ask a housewife with young children whether she works she will probably answer 'no' unless she has a paid job.

Employment can be defined as the work we do for money, whereas work is a much broader category of everything we do to keep body and soul together. Rose has calculated that more than half of our labour hours are spent not in employment but in unpaid labour in the household and community.[1] Understanding the difference between work and employment may be crucially important for the future because it is likely that there will never again be enough employment to go round, but there will always be ample work. If the barriers between work and employment were broken down and if work rather than employment were rewarded with income and status then the whole problem of unemployment might disappear. I will return to this theme.

But the main theme of this book is not the future of work but rather unemployment and health. It is 15 years since unemployment rose above a million in Britain for the first time since the Second World War, and yet only now are health workers and health authorities beginning to wake up to the profound implications for health of mass unemployment. The studies of the 1930s are having to be rediscovered and the lessons from them are having to be relearnt. Some health workers, indeed, are unwilling to accept that unemployment is anything to do with them. In response to the articles that I published in the *British Medical Journal*, Dr J. W. Maltby, a general practitioner from Tiverton, wrote:[2]

Unemployment is a political problem, a socioeconomic problem, and not a medical problem . . . It is rather like drug addiction in this respect. It is a domestic disaster, a family tragedy, but not a national tragedy—and not a medical matter, though it may become one. If doctors accept it as a medical matter they assume responsibility for it and are blamed when things do not go according to plan. We get enough of this without asking for it.

I quote Dr Maltby because I think that many doctors and other health workers might agree with him, although most would hesitate to write to the *British Medical Journal* to say so. Dr Maltby gives various unsatisfactory and unconvincing reasons why he thinks doctors should have nothing to do with unemployment, but his poorest reason is his final one—cowardice. Doctors assume responsibility for many difficult problems that are not easily soluble—motor neurone disease (a progressive muscular paralysis that eventually kills) is one that springs to mind. Dr Maltby would surely not advocate abandoning patients with motor neurone disease for fear of being blamed 'when things do not go according to plan'. Ironically, doctors probably can do much more to alleviate and even 'cure' the ill health generated by unemployment than they can to help those with motor neurone disease.

In contrast to Dr Maltby, I think that doctors, other health workers, and health authorities must take responsibility for the harm that unemployment does to health. Firstly, because unemployment is strongly associated with poor health and because there is good evidence that unemployment itself causes some of that ill health. And here I am using the narrow working definition of health that doctors and other health workers use but rarely explicitly define—that is, an absence of measurable disease. The broader definition of health adopted in many other cultures would often include having a job as part of being healthy. The World Health Organization defines health as complete physical, mental and social well-being, and thus again those who wanted employment but did not have it would by definition not be enjoying full health.

My second reason for believing that health workers must recognize the link between unemployment and poor health is that, even if they fail to recognize it, their patients will present them with health problems that are caused or compounded by unemployment. Thirdly, doctors, health workers, and health authorities can do something to alleviate those problems.

But health workers have been criticized for campaigning on issues like seat belts, smoking, alcohol, and nuclear war. Will they not stumble into even more trouble by making statements on an issue so politically sensitive as unemployment? Isn't unemployment more an economic and political problem rather than a medical one? Or will we eventually see a report from the Royal College of Physicians on unemployment and health? I think that we might. Unemployment is far too important an issue to be left to economists, and already there is a substantial body of research on how unemployment harms health. This information is, however, scattered through a variety of disciplines—including psychology, sociology, economics, history, literature, journalism, and medicine—and it has not had the prominence it deserves. The aim of this book is to bring together this scattered material.

> It is only when you lodge in the streets where nobody has a job, where getting a job seems about as probable as owning an aeroplane and much less probable than winning fifty pounds in the Football Pool, that you begin to grasp the changes that are being worked in our civilisation.
>
> GEORGE ORWELL *The Road to Wigan Pier*
> [London: Victor Gollancz, 1937]

Over 13 per cent of the British workforce is registered unemployed and seeking work, which means more than three million people; and more than a million have been unemployed for a year or longer. The number of people officially recorded as unemployed has more than doubled since the present government first came to power in 1979. There are, however, various ways of measuring the number of unemployed people, and the methods used in Britain have been varied many times in the recent past. Almost invariably the new method has produced a lower figure. In some ways the figures undoubtedly underestimate the 'true' number of unemployed: they do not include the many people, particularly women and those looking for part-time employment, who do not register as unemployed even though they want a job. The 'true' number of unemployed may thus be over four million.[3] The figure may also be an overestimate as it includes people who are simply between jobs, some who are voluntarily unemployed (probably only 12 per cent of those counted, a very much smaller number than is popularly imagined), and some who are 'unemployable'. The notion of somebody being 'unemployable' is not very useful, however, as in the right circumstances almost anybody can do something. It is also important to

> I never do any shopping, or housework, or washing or cleaning. The wife does it all. We eat meat once a week at mam and dad's. My main meal is beans and a beefburger, or a fry up. I go for a pint when the giro comes, and on Fridays I play in a darts match, and every two or three months we both go out. We live in a flat and there's no garden, so we always get on each others nerves. I get depressed and just sit and sulk, it's never physical but we shout a lot. The two kids are small so they get on my nerves. I just generally have the feeling that I'm about to blow my brains out, thinking is this it?
>
> BEATRIX CAMPBELL[35] A 22-year-old former fitter
> quoted in *Wigan Pier Revisited* [London: Virago, 1984]

realize that there is still considerable turnover in employment—about 400 000 people each month start a new job—and that there are almost as many people employed now as ever before—over 26 million. The labour force has increased as the population has grown and as more women seek paid employment, and this trend is continuing: the official estimate is that the labour force will increase by about 830 000 between 1984 and 1991.[4]

Although I will frequently use the word 'unemployed' in this book without qualification, the unemployed are not a homogeneous group: some people are simply between jobs, while others have been unemployed for years, have never worked, and maybe never will.

1,000 chase job working on tip

More than 900 men and women have applied for a vacancy as a rubbish dump attendant in Sheffield which has 47,000 unemployed.

Council officials said they were 'staggered' by the response to advertisements for the £144-a-week job. The work entails sorting rubbish at inner city domestic disposal units.

David Blunkett, Labour leader of the city council, said the response refuted the claim that there were plenty of jobs around which people would not do.

The Independent Saturday 13 December 1986, p. 1, column 6
(By permission of the Editor)

The consequences are clearly very different for these different groups. Furthermore, the young, the old, the unskilled, the single, men with large families, the disabled, the socially disadvantaged, and members of ethnic minorities are all over-represented among the unemployed. The unemployed are also concentrated in depressed industrial areas and inner cities. But compared with the 1930s regional differences in unemployment rates are greatly reduced, and in the past few years as unemployment has increased rapidly the variation in rates between skilled and unskilled has decreased. Unemployment is not simply a problem of particular people in particular places.[3]

The positive association between unemployment and a variety of measures of ill health is clear. What is less clear is how that association arises: does unemployment itself cause a deterioration in health; or are the sick most likely to become unemployed; or does the association between unemployment and poor health arise because unemployment leads to poverty, which we well know to be associated with poor health; or are unemployment and poor health both associated with other factors such as low socioeconomic status, poorer education, and worse housing conditions? These are not mutually exclusive hypotheses (although some reports on unemployment and health give that impression), and all are true to some degree. But we cannot be sure of the degree of truth of each hypothesis, and nor can we be confident about the strength of the association between unemployment and ill health. Brenner, for instance, has estimated that unemployment in Britain may be associated with tens of thousands of premature deaths,[5, 6] while Gravelle[7] is unconvinced that unemployment causes any premature death, and Scott-Samuel opts for a 'conservative' figure of 3000 a year.[8]

The evidence linking unemployment with poor mental health is much stronger than that linking it with poor physical health.[9] In

---

Nothing to do with time; nothing to spend; nothing to do tomorrow nor the day after; nothing to wear; can't get married. A living corpse; a unit of the spectral army of the three million lost men.

WALTER GREENWOOD *Love on the Dole*
[Harmondsworth: Penguin, 1969 (First published 1933)]

most surveys about a fifth of the unemployed report a deterioration in their mental health since becoming unemployed, and the longer they have been without work the more likely they are to report a deterioration.[9-11] Importantly, however, about 5 per cent of people report an improvement in their mental health—some because they have escaped from miserable jobs, but others because they have found positive aspects to unemployment.[12]

In addition to these self-reported changes in mental health, many studies have measured the mental health of the unemployed using the standardized questionnaires that are now of great importance in psychological and psychiatric research. These studies have consistently shown that the mental health of those out of work is poorer than that of the employed.[9] The unemployed tend to be more anxious, depressed, unhappy, dissatisfied, neurotic, and worried, they have lower confidence and self-esteem, and they sleep worse than the employed. That many of the unemployed should be miserable is hardly a surprise, but these questionnaires are measuring more than misery. The widely used general health questionnaire, for instance, measures a person's probability of being a psychiatric case. More than half of 401 unemployed 16- to 24-year-olds given the general health questionnaire in Australia were considered to be 'probable cases of psychiatric disorder', and 47 of a weighted subsample of 72 examined by a psychiatrist were classed as cases.[13]

But the evidence associating unemployment with full-blown psychosis is weak.[9,14] This may be partly because the association has not been much studied (psychologists have done much more work than psychiatrists). What has been studied extensively is the link between unemployment and suicide and deliberate self-injury (often called parasuicide). Platt found 156 relevant studies, and they consistently show that the unemployed are over-represented among those who kill or deliberately injure themselves and that suicide and parasuicide rates are higher among the unemployed than among the employed.[15] Studies that follow large groups through time also show more unemployment and job instability among those who kill and deliberately injure themselves, and in almost all countries studied, unemployment and suicide and parasuicide rates change together over time.

None of these studies is capable of proving that of itself unemployment leads to suicide or deliberate self-injury. But unemployment itself has been proved to cause a deterioration in measured mental health. Banks and Jackson gave the general health questionnaire to more than a 1000 16-year-olds in Leeds before and after they left school.[16] They showed not only that those who became unemployed scored higher on the general health questionnaire but also that the two groups had scores that were not significantly different when they were still at school—thus it cannot be argued, as it can with most studies of unemployment and health, that unemployment might have been associated with poorer mental health because those with the poorer health had more difficulty finding jobs. Another study by the same group has also shown that the score of the unemployed on the general health questionnaire fell sharply when they got jobs.[17]

Research into unemployment and mental health has moved into the stage of looking for mechanisms and working out who among the unemployed is most severely harmed. The fact that research into unemployment and mental health is superior to that into physical health (and I recognize that this is a somewhat false dichotomy) may reflect the fact that psychological studies are easier to do than physical ones in these circumstances, that psychologists and social scientists have taken more initiatives than doctors, and that even with an inadequate social security system the psyche of the unemployed is more harmed than their bodies.

From her studies of the unemployed in the 1930s, Jahoda produced hypotheses about what it is about employment that matters in addition to financial reward[18] (although possibly loss of income matters more than anything else).[9] Employment imposes a time structure on the day, provides social contact outside the family, gives a purpose and sense of achieving something with others, assigns social status, and requires regularity. Warr has added to this list: the unemployed lose the 'traction' of employment—the way it pulls you along and means you do more on Mondays than Sundays; they have a smaller scope for making big decisions and less chance of developing new skills; and, finally, the unemployed suffer frequent humiliations and lose social status.[9]

The usefulness of teasing out these mechanisms of how unemployment hurts is that it may allow ways of reducing the poor mental health of the unemployed, even in a society where high unemployment is likely to continue. The same can be said for studies of who among the unemployed suffers most; these show that the middle-aged tend to be more harmed than those who are younger or older, which may relate to the unsurprising finding that the more somebody wants a job the more his mental health is likely to suffer during unemployment.[9] Other groups who suffer disproportionately are the poorest, those who do the least, and the 'vulnerable': mothers, and particularly young mothers, seem to be protected from the psychological distress of unemployment.

Studies on how unemployment affects physical health cannot match the sophistication of the psychological studies, and many of those that have been done concentrate on death. Furthermore, most have used data for whole populations over long periods of time and have used complex mathematical techniques to search for associations between measures of performance of the economy—including unemployment—and measures of health such as overall and infant mortality. These studies are called aggregate studies or time-series analyses, and, although they were for a time at the centre of the debate over unemployment and health, they have now diminished in importance.

Singer used aggregate analyses in the 1930s to show correlations between unemployment and maternal and infant mortality,[19] and Morris and Titmuss extended Singer's work in the 1940s to show correlations between unemployment and deaths from rheumatic heart disease in 83 county boroughs in England and Wales from 1927–38, even after controlling for poverty and overcrowding.[20] These studies have since been severely criticized,[21] as have the more recent studies of Brenner in which he has shown a relation between economic instability and mortality in the United States, England and Wales,[5] and Scotland. His own data for England and Wales were reworked, and no statistically significant relation was found between unemployment and mortality.[22] Brenner retorted that his model had not been applied properly in the new analysis.[23]

There are several problems with these aggregate studies. They can show only correlation, not causation; because they measure mortality in whole populations, they cannot sort out the mortality of the unemployed from that of the employed; minor procedural changes in the methods may produce dramatically different results; they are all studies of the past and so may not be relevant to the present; and they cannot tease out the effects of unemployment from those of poverty, availability of health services, changes in diet, etc.[9]

Much better data can be obtained from longitudinal studies that follow a defined population through changes in employment status and see what happens to particular individuals. Sadly, although unemployment began to increase dramatically in Britain more than five years ago, no study was ever set up to examine specifically the effect of unemployment on mortality—or, indeed, on any other measure of health. Instead, clever use has had to be made of data from studies set up for other purposes, and the cleverest of these opportunistic studies has been that derived from the longitudinal study of the Office of Population Censuses and Surveys that follows up a one per cent sample of the population of England and Wales from the 1971 census.

Moser *et al.* found that the standardized mortality ratio in 1971–81 of the 5861 men who were seeking work or waiting to take up a job in the week before the census was 136 (95 per cent confidence limits 122–152).[24] The ratio was raised for all age groups and was over 200 in those aged 35–44. The authors calculated that some of this increased mortality among the unemployed was due to unequal socioeconomic distribution, but in all social classes the mortality of the unemployed was higher than that of the employed. Moser *et al.* also were very ingenious in trying to work out whether this excess mortality among the unemployed was due to the sick being more likely to become unemployed. They hypothesized that if this was the case then mortality would be higher in the whole group in the first half of the decade, and this was not so. They also hypothesized that if it was unemployment itself that caused the extra deaths then the wives of the men might be affected, and they found a standardized mortality ratio of 120 (95 per cent confidence limits, 102–139) among the 2906 wives.

This is the most outstanding study yet on mortality among the unemployed, but because of the complexity of their hypotheses and their large sampling variations the authors were unable to be completely confident that unemployment itself kills. They also warned against using the data to draw conclusions about unemployment in the 1980s. It might have been that unemployment in 1971, when the overall rate was very much lower than in the 1980s, was a very different experience. Perhaps it was more lethal then and perhaps any

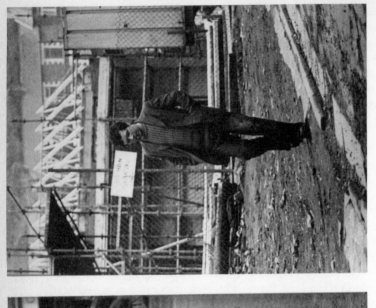

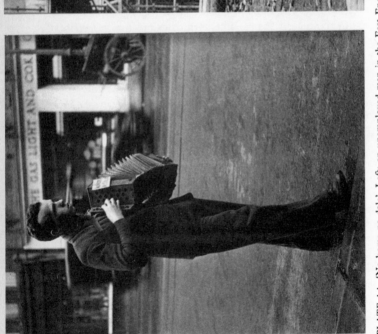

PLATE 1.1 'No home no dole'. Left: an unemployed man in the East End of London in the 1930s (photographed by Edith Tudor Wright, copyright W. Suschitzsky). Right: an unemployed man in South Wales in the 1980s (photograph by John Sturrock, copyright Report).

effect that selected out the sick for unemployment would have been much more important than when unemployment became a much more common experience. Early analysis from data collected in 1981 shows, however, very similar trends to those from 1971.[25]

Far more limited are the studies of physical health that have used end points other than death. One often-quoted study was of 113 men who lost their jobs when two manufacturing plants in Michigan closed in 1967.[26] The study was controlled, and the men were followed from 4 to 7 weeks before the plants closed until two years after: they were interviewed several times, kept a health diary, and had their blood pressure and serum cholesterol and uric acid concentrations measured. The design of this study thus meant that it had the potential to produce convincing results, but it did not. It did suggest that the changes in employment caused more problems than unemployment itself, but Cook and Shaper are fair when they say that the results of this study are less interesting than the methods.[27] It was intended as a pilot study but tragically has never been repeated with larger numbers and better measures.

The British Regional Heart Study, which is looking at variations in heart disease in 24 medium-sized British towns, has also been used to produce information on unemployment and health and has shown higher rates of bronchitis, chronic obstructive lung disease, and ischaemic heart disease among the unemployed than among the employed.[28] But many of the unemployed said that they had become unemployed because of poor health, and only very limited conclusions are possible. The same goes for the Department of Health and Social Security cohort study[29] and the United Kingdom Training Survey,[30] both of which have produced unconvincing information on the health of the unemployed—chiefly because neither was primarily designed for that purpose. The only study that was sponsored specifically by the DHSS to look at the health of the unemployed was that by Fagin.[31] He looked at 22 families in depth and produced fine descriptions of their plight, but his study does not allow conclusions on whether unemployment causes ill health.

One new study has, however, produced convincing data on how unemployment affects consultation rates in general practice. It came surprisingly from a small town in Wiltshire—Calne.[32] One of the local general practitioners, Dr Norman Beale, identified the records of the families of 80 men and 49 women who had lost their jobs when the local sausage factory closed and matched them closely with controls who had not lost their jobs. He and a statistician, Susan Nethercott, looked at consultation rates from five years before the factory closed and are planning to carry on the study until five years after the closure. They found a statistically significant 20 per cent increase in consultation rate for the families of those eventually made redundant compared with controls from two years before the factory closed, a time when the workers first knew that closure was likely. They also found a 60 per cent increase in referrals to hospital out-patients.

This study has the great advantages of being longitudinal and controlled, of starting well before the factory closed, and of including whole families. The disadvantage is that so far the data cover only consultations, and patients have many reasons for visiting their doctors—not all of them include clearly defined physical or mental illness. Further analysis will show why these patients consulted.

The Calne study has added considerably to what is otherwise very thin data on how the health of the families of the unemployed might be harmed. Unemployment is associated with high divorce rates, child abuse and neglect, wife battering, unwanted pregnancies, abortions, reduced birthweight of babies, increased perinatal and infant mortality, reduced growth in children, and increased morbidity in wives and children. But for none of these associations can we be confident that unemployment itself is the cause.

Why when we have more than three million people unemployed do we have so little information on how unemployment affects physical health? Some people whom I spoke to thought that the government had deliberately discouraged research on unemployment and health because it did not want any data produced that might make continuing with present economic policies more difficult. Certainly I was told by a reliable source that in Scotland the government word went round saying that research into unemployment and health was not a priority; and this could not be argued on the grounds either that we know enough about unemployment and health or that it is an unimportant subject. I heard of at least two other cases from England where applications for grants to do research into unemployment and health had been rejected more on political than scientific grounds.

But others I spoke to subscribed less to this conspiracy theory and more to the idea that the leaders of health workers had been slow to wake up to the importance of unemployment to health (and maybe they are not awake yet). One important hindrance may be that the departments of health are unenthusiastic about sponsoring research into unemployment because that is a matter for the Department of Employment, and in its turn the Department of Employment does not think that it has any responsibility to sponsor health research. Others think that there is not much point in researching unemployment and health because all that could be done as a result would be to argue for less unemployment, which everybody wants anyway but appears 'hard' to achieve.

This last argument is wrong on at least two grounds: firstly, a fuller understanding of the damage done to the unemployed might mean that much more weight would be given to such facts when political and economic decisions were being made on employment; secondly, much can be done—other than the creation of new jobs by government—to alleviate the sufferings of the unemployed. The Unemployment and Health Study Group has produced plans on how to prevent the health consequences of unemployment and on how they can be modified by the health services and other agencies.[33] The first thing that can be done is to reduce poverty among the unemployed by raising benefits, but at the moment the government seems set on doing the opposite. Another possibility is to change the rules so that the unemployed can do a little paid work without losing their benefits. A further ploy would be to share out the work that is available by creating job-sharing agreements, shortening working days and weeks, offering early retirement, longer holidays, and sabbaticals, and by rotating periods of worklessness. In the past these sorts of measures have been used most in industries where unemployment is looming rather than throughout the labour market, and for them to become widespread may require changes in the way that most people think about employment.

Health authorities and individual health workers can also do much to counter the harmful effects of unemployment on health. Table 1.1 shows what health authorities might do, and Table 1.2 shows what individual health workers might do. A survey that I conducted with a medical student, Christiane Harris, surprised me by showing that many health authorities are now putting together a response to

TABLE 1.1. Steps that might be taken by health authorities to respond to the health problems of unemployment

---

(1) Monitoring unemployment and its effects on health in your area
(2) Relaying this information to staff
(3) Taking unemployment into account when allocating resources
(4) Creating jobs and work—either on your own initiative or together with the Manpower Services Commission
(4) Encouraging and training staff to familiarize themselves with facilities and benefits for the unemployed, and perhaps seconding some to local community initiatives
(5) Making information about facilities and benefits for the unemployed available to staff. Such facilities include:
   advisory bodies
   counselling/psychological help
   job creation schemes
   leisure/recreation schemes
   retraining/education
   practical skills (such as furniture repair and preparation of cheap but nutritious meals)
   women's groups
   youth groups
   ethnic groups
(6) Liaising with local authorities and other health authorities to ensure that efforts are not being duplicated and to assess whether you could do anything to further their efforts
(7) Targeting your responses at those most in need

---

unemployment's effects on health. More details of this response will be presented later.

In the long term, however, the answer to unemployment may be for us to learn to value unpaid work as much as employment. Handy foresees a future in which people might be given a basic income that did not depend on being in employment. People could then if they chose spend much of their time doing unpaid work, but they would also be free to top up their income with employment. This extra work would probably be done much more flexibly, and overall people would spend less time in employment and would propor-tionately have a smaller income. Both employment and money would be shared out. In this way an age-old dream of freeing people from dreary toil might be achieved without creating a vast scrap heap of unemployed, unwanted, unhappy people. In such a community

TABLE 1.2. What health workers can do about unemployment and health

- Recognise problems in their patients caused by unemployment
- Know their patients' occupational histories
- Refer their patients for advice on benefits
- Know of national and local initiatives to help the unemployed and so be able to refer patients
- Work locally to make people aware of the health consequences of unemployment and so help to reduce the stigma of unemployment
- Consider organizing employment schemes either alone or with the Manpower Services Commission

that valued both work and employment health would not be damaged by unemployment. Indeed, 'unemployment' as we know it would be gone.

References

1. Rose, R. *Getting by in three economies*. Glasgow: Centre for the Study of Public Policy, University of Strathclyde, 1983.

2. Maltby, J.W. Occupationless health. *Br. Med. J.* 1986; **292**: 488.

3. Hawkins, K. *Unemployment*. Harmondsworth: Penguin, 1984.

4. Anonymous. Labour force outlook for Great Britain. *Employment Gazette* 1985; July: 255-64.

5. Brenner, M.H. Mortality and the national economy: a review, and the experience of England and Wales. *Lancet* 1979; **ii**: 568-73.

6. Brenner, M.H. Health costs and benefits of economic policy. *Int. J. Health Serv.* 1977; **7**: 581-93.

7. Gravelle, H. *Does unemployment kill?* Oxford: Nuffield Provincial Hospitals Trust, 1985.

8. Scott-Samuel, A. Unemployment and health. *Lancet* 1984; **ii**: 1464-5.

9. Warr, P. Twelve questions about unemployment and health. In: Roberts, R., Finnegan, R., Gallie, D., eds. *New approaches to economic life*. Manchester: Manchester University Press, 1985.

10. Jackson, P.R., Warr, P.B. Unemployment and psychological ill health: the moderating role of duration and age. *Psychol. Med.* 1984; **14**: 605-14.

11. Colledge, M., Bartholomew, R. *A study of the long term unemployed.* London: Manpower Services Commission, 1980.

12. Fryer, D., Payne, R. Proactive behaviour in unemployment: findings and implications. *Leisure Studies* 1984; **3**: 273-95.

13. Finlay-Jones, R., Eckhardt, B. Psychiatric disorder among the young unemployed. *Aust. N.Z. J. Psychiat.* 1981; **15**: 265-70.

14. Jaco, E.G. *The social epidemiology of mental disorders.* New York: Russell Sage Foundation, 1960.

15. Platt, S. Unemployment and suicidal behaviour: a review of the literature. *Soc. Sci. Med.* 1984; **19**: 93-115.

16. Banks, M.H., Jackson, P.R. Unemployment and risk of minor psychiatric disorder in young people: cross sectional and longitudinal evidence. *Psychol. Med.* 1982; **12**: 789-98.

17. Jackson, P.R., Stafford, E.M., Banks, M.H., Warr, P.B. *Work involvement and employment status as influences on mental health: a test of an interactional model.* Sheffield: Social and Applied Psychology Unit, University of Sheffield, 1982 (Memo 404).

18. Jahoda, M. *Employment and unemployment.* Cambridge: Cambridge University Press, 1982.

19. Singer, H. *Unemployment and health.* London: Pilgrim Trust, 1937 (Pilgrim Trust Unemployment Enquiry Interim Paper).

20. Morris, J.N., Titmuss, R.M. *Medical Officer* 1940; **2**; 69.

21. Stern, J. *Unemployment and its impact on morbidity and mortality.* London: London School of Economics Centre for Labour Economics, 1981.

22. Gravelle H.S.E., Hutchinson, G., Stern, J. Mortality and unemployment: a critique of Breener's time series analysis. *Lancet* 1981; **ii**: 675-9.

23. Brenner, M.H. Unemployment and health. *Lancet* 1981; **ii**: 874-5.

24. Moser, K.A., Fox, A.J., Jones, D.R. Unemployment and mortality in the OPCS longitudinal study. *Lancet* 1984; **ii**: 1324-9.

25. Moser, K.A., Goldblatt, P.O., Fox, A.J., Jones, D.R. Unemployment and mortality: comparison of the 1971 and 1981 longitudinal census samples. *Br. Med. J.* 1987; **294**: 86-90.

26. Kasl, S. Strategies of research on economic instability and health. *Psychol. Med.* 1982; **12**: 637-49.

27. Cook, D.G., Shaper, A.G. Unemployment and health. In: Harrington, J.M., ed. *Recent advances in occupational health*, Vol II. Edinburgh: Churchill Livingstone, 1985.

28. Cook, D.G., Cummins, R.O., Bartley, M.J., Shaper, A.G. Health of unemployed middle aged men in Great Britain. *Lancet* 1982; **i**: 1290-4.

29. Moylan, S., Millar, J., Davies, R. *For richer, for poorer? DHSS study of unemployed men*. London: HMSO, 1984.

30. Narendranathan, W., Nickell, S., Metcalf, D. *An investigation into the incidence and dynamic structure of sickness and unemployment in Britain, 1965-75*. London: London School of Economics Centre for Labour Economics, 1982. (Discussion paper 142.)

31. Fagin, L., Little, M. *The forsaken families*. Harmondsworth: Penguin, 1984.

32. Beale, N., Nethercott, S. Job loss and family morbidity: a study of factory closure. *J. R. Coll. Gen. Pract.* 1985; **280**: 510-4.

33. Unemployment and Health Study Group. *Unemployment, health, and social policy*. Leeds: Nuffield Centre for Health Services Studies, 1984.

2

A guide to the facts and figures of unemployment

IF they want to do their best by their patients doctors must, it seems, increasingly look up from their microscopes and the chests they are percussing to consider the wider world. The same goes for all health workers. So I make no apology for this guide to the extent and causes of unemployment because unemployment probably now does much more damage to health in Britain than does the tubercle bacillus. Indeed, even when considering tuberculosis John Maynard Keynes may have done as much to reduce mortality as did Robert Koch. Doctors may not be able to take their scalpels to unemployment (much as they may wish they could), but they need to understand its scope, distribution, causes, and course so that they can minister to individual patients and communities. And studies on unemployment and health make sense only when you know who the unemployed are and how long they have been without work.

About three and a third million people in Britain are officially recorded as unemployed—that is, about 13 per cent of the workforce. Over two million men are unemployed (about 16 per cent), and just under a million women (about 10 per cent). More than 1.3 million people have been unemployed for more than a year, which is about 40 per cent of the total. This proportion is likely to rise remorselessly. In addition, more than half a million people have been unemployed for three years or longer.

These figures for the number of unemployed people are derived from counting those receiving unemployment benefit, but before November 1982 the count was of the number of people registered with the Department of Employment as seeking and being capable of and available for work. This gave a figure about 6 per cent higher than the current method. Many other more minor variations have been made in the way the unemployed are defined and counted, and almost invariably these revisions reduce the overall figure.

No method can be entirely accurate, and counting the unemployed is as difficult as counting the number of 'cases' of a disease—much depends on the definitions and methods used. The official methods underestimate the true numbers of the unemployed because many people who are seeking work, particularly part-time work, do not register as unemployed and are not entitled to unemployment benefit. Estimates made from the census and the General Household Survey suggest that in the early 1970s about 245 000 people, most of them women, fell into this category.[1] Furthermore, as unemployment increases the number of people who do not register probably rises because they see no point. The Warwick Manpower Research Group has estimated that only about 71 per cent of those seeking work (78 per cent of men and 58 per cent of women) register, which, if correct, inflates the true number of unemployed to over four million.

But the conventional methods also overestimate the number of the unemployed because they include those between jobs and those who are voluntarily unemployed or effectively 'unemployable'. The Department of Employment introduced this notion of people being unemployable but at the same time warned against using it too rigidly—everybody can do something.

As Hawkins clearly argues, better measures still are the flow of people into and out of employment and the median time that people spend unemployed: even now about 400 000 people a month are stopping receiving unemployment benefit and presumably starting a job. At the same time, unfortunately, slightly more people are losing their jobs and beginning to claim benefit. Many people do not spend long on the dole: in the 1960s about half of those who lost their jobs got another one within two weeks. Daniel estimated that in 1981 about a third of those becoming unemployed got a job within a month, the median duration of unemployment being three to four months.[2]

Economists have classified unemployment into three types: frictional, structural, and cyclical. Frictional unemployment results simply from the time people spend between jobs: as there are about nine million job changes a year inevitably some people will not step straight from one job to another. Beveridge thought that up to 3 per cent of the working population at any one time might be between jobs.[3] Structural unemployment arises from a mismatch between the jobs available and the skills of the unemployed. It implies that if the unemployed learnt new skills then they would find a job in their own locality. At least some of the current unemployment is structural because there are jobs vacancies in electronics, and electrical and mechanical engineering, and for people with knowledge of the new technologies. Cyclical unemployment is caused by economic recession, and is beyond the control of individual employers and not limited to particular trades. Most of today's unemployment is cyclical.

In the past 12 years in Britain unemployment has increased roughly fivefold. Figure 2.1 shows the changes in the number of unemployed and vacancies notified to job centres (roughly a third of vacancies) between 1964 and 1985, and Fig. 2.2 shows the changes in the gap between those available for work and those working between 1964 and 1985. Some unemployment is resulting from an increase in the size of the working population, the latest government prediction being that the labour force will grow by 830 000 between 1984 and 1991, about 400 000 more than was predicted in August 1984.[4] The increase in the number of unemployed cannot have escaped anyone's attention and is now the most important issue on the political agenda.

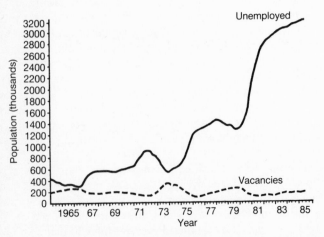

FIG. 2.1 Unemployment and vacancies recorded at employment offices (about a third of all vacancies) in the UK from 1964 to 1985.

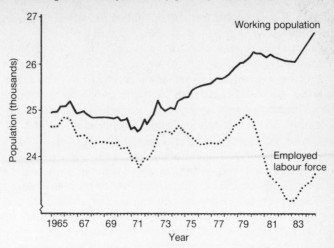

FIG. 2.2 Working population and employed labour force in UK from 1965 to 1984.

Everybody knows, too, of the depression of the interwar years. In August 1932, the nadir of the depression, 2 947 000 (23 per cent) insured workers were unemployed.[5] Knowing that about 70 per cent of workers were insured and that unemployment was lower among those not insured, we can calculate that the total number unemployed was about 3 500 000. There may thus now be more people unemployed than in the 1930s but the proportion unemployed is lower. The depression of the 1930s was, of course, international, and other countries had similar unemployment: in 1932 it was 32 per cent in the United States, 29 per cent in Australia, and 22 per cent in Canada and Sweden. Germany had more than 5.5 million unemployed in 1932.

But unemployment goes back much further than the 1930s. It existed in medieval Britain but became apparent for the first time on a large scale with the industrial revolution.[6] It reached 11 per cent in the depression of 1874–87, which was caused by the near-completion of the railways, overproduction in shipping and steel, agricultural depression, and increasing foreign competition. Both world wars saw full employment, although it took a little longer to come about in the Second World War. Between 1948 and 1966 the average number of unemployed was about 350 000, less than 2 per cent of the workforce.

Unemployment rates also vary regionally, but this variation is decreasing. In the 1930s unemployment was five times higher in Wales than in London and the South-east and three times higher in Scotland, the North-west, and the North-east. Now, as Table 2.1 shows, unemployment is about 10 per cent in London and the South-east, and 17 per cent in Wales, 16 per cent in Scotland, 16 per cent in the North-west, and 19 per cent in the North-east.[7] Northern Ireland has the highest rate at about 21 per cent. But there are also considerable variations within regions (Fig. 2.3). In Scotland, for instance, in March 1985 unemployment varied between 6.4 per cent in Aberdeen and 24.1 per cent in Cumnock and Sanquar; and in Northern Ireland, it varied from 13.9 per cent in Ballymena to 39.5 per cent in Strabane (the highest in the country). There is also variation on an even smaller scale: the London parliamentary constituency of Vauxhall, for instance, in March 1985 had 10 381 unemployed people, while the constituency of Surbiton, 15 minutes away by train, had only 1583—a difference of more than sixfold, greater than the difference between the South-east and Wales in the 1930s.

Unemployment remains an international problem, and Table 2.2 gives figures from the Department of Employment on unemployment rates in selected countries. These cannot be directly compared as different methods are used to measure unemployment, but they do show increasing unemployment all over the world. Some countries (Japan, Norway, and Sweden) have managed to keep their unemployment to about 3 per cent, and only four (Belgium, the

TABLE 2.1. Regional variation in percentage unemployment rate

Region (Per cent)	Unemployment	Region (Per cent)	Unemployment %
Northern Ireland	20.7	Yorkshire and Humberside	14.9
North	18.8	East Midlands	12.5
Wales	16.5	South-west	11.6
North-west	16.2	Greater London	10.6
Scotland	15.5	East Anglia	10.3
West Midlands	15.4	South East (including London)	9.9

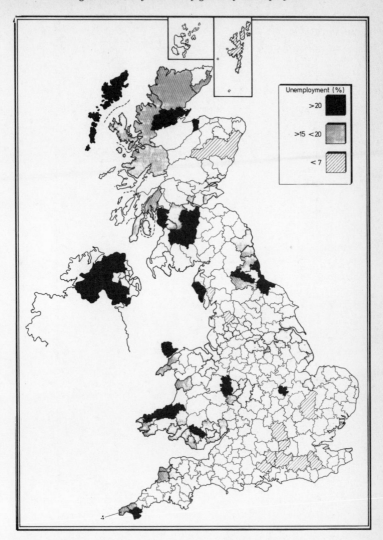

FIG. 2.3 Variations in percentage unemployment by 'travel to work' area. Most areas (white) fall in the range 7-15 per cent, but 12 areas have rates below 7 per cent and almost 40 areas (including most of Northern Ireland) have rates above 20 per cent (see key).

TABLE 2.2. Percentage unemployment in selected countries from 1980 to 1985

	United Kingdom	Australia	Austria	Belgium	Canada	Denmark	France	Germany	Greece
1980	6.9	5.6	1.9	11.7	6.6	6.9	7.6	3.6	2.1
1981	10.4	4.8	2.4	14.2	6.9	9.0	9.3	5.2	2.4
1982	12.1	6.8	3.7	16.6	10.0	9.6	10.5	7.4	2.9
1983	12.8	9.6	4.5	18.3	11.0	10.5	10.7	9.2	3.6
1984	13.1	8.9	4.6	18.6	10.7	10.3	12.1	9.2	4.1
1985 (2nd quarter)	13.4	8.4	4.2	17.3	10.3	10.9*	11.9	9.0	4.0

	Irish Republic	Italy	Japan	Netherlands	Norway	Spain	Sweden	Switzerland	United States
1980	7.9	7.8	1.9	6.7	1.1	10.6	1.9	0.2	6.5
1981	9.9	8.8	2.1	10.3	1.4	13.0	2.4	0.2	7.1
1982	12.1	10.5	2.3	14.0	2.1	15.5	3.1	0.5	9.1
1983	14.9	12.0	2.7	17.2	3.2	18.3	3.4	0.9	9.1
1984	16.5	13.0	2.7	17.6	3.3	20.6	3.1	1.1	7.3
1985 (2nd quarter)	17.5	12.8	2.8*	15.9	3.3*	22.1*	3.1*	1.1*	7.1

*Values for first quarter, not second.

Netherlands, Spain, and the Irish Republic) have higher rates than Britain.

Unemployment does not occur randomly in the population. The young, the old, the unskilled, the single, men with large families, the disabled, the socially disadvantaged, members of ethnic minorities, and those who have been to prison are over-represented among the unemployed, and particularly among the long-term unemployed.[1, 6] Nevertheless, since 1979, when unemployment began to grow very rapidly, all sorts of groups—including the skilled and those in the middle of their working lives—have been much more affected.[1, 6] Just as the differential between employment in the north and south is fading, so is that between the skilled and the unskilled. As Hawkins puts it, unemployment is not a problem of 'particular people in particular places', and programmes to increase employment and lessen the consequences of unemployment cannot be concentrated on particular areas and groups—they are needed by all.[1]

One important group which is over-represented among the unemployed is that of people over 55: they are more likely to be made redundant and also find it more difficult to get another job. Daniel has said that age is of 'overwhelming' importance compared with skill.[8] In the 1970s a third of those who had been unemployed for more than a year were over 55, but as unemployment has grown the proportion has fallen to nearer a fifth (although the absolute numbers have, of course, grown) (Fig. 2.4).

At the other end of the age range, those under 20 are more likely to be unemployed than those who are older, and as unemployment rises it rises disproportionately among the young. Between April 1979 and April 1982 total male unemployment increased from 6.6 to 15 per cent, while among men under 20 (excluding school leavers) it increased from 9.1 to 25 per cent—a ratio of 1:1.9.[1] For women over the same period the ratio was even higher—1:2.4. Furthermore, although the young were once more likely than older people to get new jobs, this is changing: in July 1977 only 7.5 per cent of those under 25 had been unemployed for more than a year but by July 1982 it was 21 per cent. In January 1985 there were 365 000 people under 25 who had been unemployed for more than a year. The worry is that some of these young people may remain unemployed for ever: one undisputed fact about unemployment is that the longer you are without a job the less likely you are to get one.

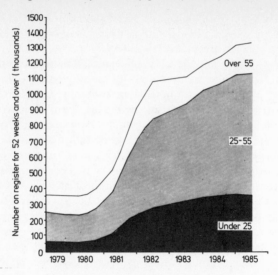

FIG. 2.4 Numbers unemployed for more than a year, by age.

Among the young unemployed it is the unskilled and the un-
qualified who are most likely to be unemployed, but this is true for
all age groups. A Survey by the Manpower Services Commission of
1698 people who had been unemployed for more than a year showed
that 59 per cent were unskilled or semiskilled and 77 per cent had no
formal qualifications.[9] Long-term unemployment among unskilled
men is likely to increase along with the shift from manufacturing to
service industries because, although most unskilled manufacturing
jobs are done by men, most unskilled jobs in the service industries
are done by women.

Unemployment among ethnic minorities seems to be worse than
among the population generally, although figures do not so easily
come to hand. Unemployment rates tend to be higher in areas where
ethnic minorities are concentrated, and Hawkins quotes figures
showing that between February 1977 and August 1982 in Bradford
unemployment among whites increased by 240 per cent and among
Asians by 330 per cent.[1]

It will come as no surprise to anybody that disabled people are
much more likely to be unemployed than the general population. In

1983 there were 56 800 registered and 90 700 unregistered disabled people who were suitable for ordinary employment and looking for jobs; 49 700 (88 per cent) of the former and 76 500 (84 per cent) of the latter were unemployed.[10] The latest figures show that more disabled people are now employed—49 per cent of those registered disabled and half of those unregistered.

In the past the long-term unemployed were very different from the short-term unemployed, but these differences are beginning to break down. The Manpower Services Commission study, published in 1980, showed that almost two-thirds of the long-term unemployed were semiskilled or unskilled and also confirmed the national figure that about a third were over 55.[9] In addition, nearly two-thirds lived in areas of high unemployment; many came from construction, manufacturing, and basic industries (and many of these had been made redundant); more than a third had some handicap or illness (13 per cent were registered disabled); and some had specific problems—poor work records, illiteracy, domestic problems, or a prison record. A survey done today would find that many of these factors have been diluted—not because these disadvantaged people have got jobs but because they have been joined by many more without any disadvantages.

One important question that must be considered is, 'How many people choose to be unemployed?' The idea that many people do make such a choice—because they are 'shirkers' or are better off receiving social security—has enough advocates to be worth dismissing. Firstly, all surveys of the unemployed show that the majority want a job and think of unemployment as bad. In Daniel's study almost three quarters said that for them being out of work was 'bad' or 'very bad.'[8] The Manpower Services Commission study found that most respondents wanted to be working and that only 8 per cent were not looking for jobs—this was usually because of their age.[9] These were all people who had been unemployed for a year or longer, and, as the report says: 'There comes a point where people can no longer sustain their motivation in the face of continued rejection, heightened awareness of their own shortcomings, disillusion with job finding services, belief that all available options have been covered, and a knowledge that jobs are scarce anyway.'

Secondly, very few people are better off financially when unemployed. The Department of Health and Social Security's study of a cohort of men who became unemployed in 1978 shows that about 7 per cent of men were as well or better off when unemployed than when employed.[11] But more than a third had an income less than half of that when they were working. Fitting these results that show a very few people are financially better off when unemployed together with studies showing that a small percentage of people enjoy better physical and mental health when they become unemployed and take a positive attitude to not having a paid job,[12] we may conclude that some people may choose to be unemployed— at least for a while. In periods like the 1960s when there was little unemployment this group may have accounted for a higher proportion of the unemployed, but now they constitute only a small proportion. The vast majority are worse off, dislike being unemployed, and want a job desparately.

I want now to consider briefly the causes of unemployment, but in doing so I stand on the edge of the inexplicable, the incomprehensible, and the controversial. Although I am not frightened of the last, I am wary of the other two factors, and so I will say little and step lightly.

Worldwide recession and a change in technology so that fewer people are needed to produce more goods and services are the two main factors that have led to increasing unemployment. Although one factor (the recession) may go away, the other will not. Sherman has estimated that three out of four current jobs could be automated by the turn of the century.[13] The increase in the number of people seeking jobs is also important. The increase is partly caused by an increase in the population and partly by more women seeking employment. The International Labour Organization estimates that one billion new jobs will have to be created by the year 2000 if there is to be full employment worldwide.[14] The director general of the organization has concluded: 'It has to be fully understood that there will be no situation of full employment if we are speaking of conventional employment.'[14]

These factors have been at work in all 'mature' economies, but unemployment has increased particularly rapidly in Britain (Fig. 2.5). Its manufacturing industries, which used to supply most of the jobs, have contracted sharply. This has something to do with low 'productivity', meaning not that Britain is full of lazy workers but rather that the quantity of goods and services produced in relation to the amount of labour, capital, energy, and entrepreneurial

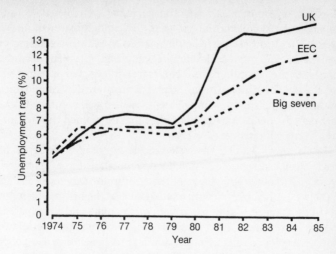

FIG. 2.5 Increase in unemployment rate in UK, countries of the EEC, and the 'big seven' (United States, United Kingdom, France, West Germany, Japan, Canada, Italy).

skills, etc. is low. Particularly important have been the failures to invest in new technology, exploit export opportunities, design products that are wanted, and conduct good industrial relations. Hawkins makes the crude calculation that if productivity in Britain were as high as that in West Germany then 7.5 million jobs could disappear for the same output.[1] Many economists have argued that the present government's economic measures have increased unemployment in Britain relative to that in other European countries: Pollard has claimed that 1.5 million willing workers owe their unemployment to the government.[15]

The poor productivity in Britain in relation to competitors is something that economic historians have observed since Victorian times, and Britain's failure cannot be explained away in purely economic terms—it has something to do with British society and culture. This is a somewhat pessimistic conclusion because British society and culture must be even more difficult to change than the British economy.

Barring the introduction of a radical policy specifically designed to cut unemployment few forecasters imagine that unemployment will fall much in Britain this decade. Indeed, it may well increase because the labour force will continue to grow, reflecting high birth rates in the early 1960s (those entering the market) and low rates during the First World War (those leaving). In addition, the manufacturing industries are continuing to contract without much expansion elsewhere. The University of Warwick Institute for Employment Research predicts that unemployment for men will continue to rise, reaching 18.5 per cent by 1990,[16] while that for women will decline a little, reaching 7 per cent by 1990.

Most of those who are interested in the future of work agree that there will never again be as much employment as there has been in the past. As Handy, the doyen of these futurologists, has explained, not only has unemployment increased but also the nature of employment has changed.[17] Compared with our parents and grandparents we start employment later, finish when we are younger, work fewer hours in a week, and take longer holidays. A generation ago people would expect to work for 100 000 hours in a lifetime (47 hours a week for 47 weeks a year for 47 years), but now even those with jobs are down to 50 000 (37 hours a week for 37 weeks a year for 37 years). Some professionals may adopt yet another pattern and work long hours for fewer years, and some others—pop singers or sports stars—may work round the clock for just a few years. But whatever the pattern, the trend for the total number of employment hours to decline is likely to continue. This might or might not go with higher unemployment, depending on whether or not the hours available are shared out.

Unemployment, as well as being damaging for the individual, is expensive to the country. In February 1982 a political decision was taken not to publish Treasury estimates of the cost to the Exchequer of unemployment, and since then estimates have had to be unofficial. One study commissioned by BBC North East estimates that unemployment costs the British Exchequer £20 billion, or £6300 for each unemployed person.[18] The Institute for Fiscal Studies produced an estimate for the House of Lords Select Committee on Unemployment of £4495 for each unemployed person in 1981-2.[19] The committee upped this figure to a 'reasonable' estimate of £5000, giving an overall figure of £15 billion.[20] None of these estimates includes lost production or other indirect costs that might arise—such as that to the National Health Service from the extra health problems of the unemployed. Nor do they include the cost to the unemployed themselves.

Sinfield and Fraser, who did the work for the BBC, were conservative in their estimates. They put the cost of benefits paid to the unemployed at £7140 million—£1760 million for unemployment benefit, £4640 million for supplementary and housing benefit, and another £740 million for men over 60 who are no longer required to register for benefits and for the unemployed in Northern Ireland. In addition, there are government costs of £300 million from the redundancy fund, which bears almost half of the costs of the state scheme, giving a total of £7440 million. The cost of lost revenue is put by Sinfield and Fraser at between £12 465 million and £12 990 million—£5690 million from lost income tax, £5200 million from lost national insurance contributions, and £2100 million from lost indirect taxes (or £1575 million if the unemployed are using up their savings). Sinfield and Fraser also made estimates of costs to local authorities, which include free school meals, higher student awards, lost revenue on buses, and increased costs for pupils staying on into sixth forms, careers services, and youth training schemes. Using data from Cleveland, they arrived at a figure of £490 for each unemployed person.

All of this £20 billion would not be saved if unemployment were suddenly eliminated, as it costs money to create jobs, but Sinfield and Fraser calculate that if unemployment were now 5.4 per cent, which it was when the Conservatives first came into office, then the cost to the exchequer would be £7.5-£12.5 billion less than it is now.

References

1. Hawkins, K. *Unemployment*. Harmondsworth: Penguin, 1984.

2. Daniel, W.W. Why is high unemployment still somehow acceptable? *New Society* 1981; March.

3. Beveridge, W. *Full employment in a free society*. London: George Allen and Unwin, 1960.

4. Anonymous. Labour force outlook for Great Britain. *Employment Gazette* 1985; July: 255-64.

5. Dearle, N.B. Unemployment. In: Law, M.D., ed. *Chamber's Encyclopadia* Vol XIV. London: George Newnes, 1950.

34   *A guide to the facts and figures of unemployment*

6. Sinfield, A. *What unemployment means*. Oxford: Martin Robertson, 1981.

7. Anonymous. Labour market data. *Employment Gazette* 1985; April: S1–S64.

8. Daniel, W.W. *A national survey of the unemployed*. London: Political and Economic Planning, 1974.

9. Colledge, M., Bartholomew, R. *A study of the long term unemployed*. Sheffield: Manpower Services Commission, 1980.

10. Anonymous. Disabled jobseekers. *Employment Gazette* 1985; April: 163.

11. Moylan, S., Millar, J., Davies, R. *For richer, for poorer? DHSS study of unemployed men*. London: HMSO, 1984.

12. Fryer, D., Payne, R. Proactive behaviour in unemployment: findings and implications. *Leisure Studies* 1984; **3**: 273-95.

13. Sherman, B. *Working at leisure*. London: Methuen, 1986.

14. International Labour Organization. Quoted in: Swift R. Useful work or useless toil. *New Internationalist* 1986; December: 4-6.

15. Pollard, S. Economic management 1974–84: an overview. *Catalyst* 1985; Spring.

16. University of Warwick Institute for Employment Research. *Review of the Economy and Employment*. Coventry: Institute for Economic Research, 1985.

17. Handy, C. *The future of work*. Oxford: Basil Blackwell, 1986.

18. Sinfield, A., Fraser, N. *The real cost of unemployment*. Newcastle: BBC North East, 1985.

19. Dilnot, A.W., Morris, C.N. The Exchequer costs of unemployment. *Fiscal Studies* 1981; **2**.

20. House of Lords Select Committee on Unemployment. *Report*. London: HMSO, 1982.

3

'Please never let it happen again'
Lessons on unemployment from the 1930s

We entered Marienthal as scientists; we leave it with only one desire: that the tragic opportunity for such an inquiry may not recur in our time.

THESE words were written by Austrian researchers who had spent months living and studying in Marienthal, a small town close to Vienna that had only one factory. When the factory closed almost everybody became unemployed. Their study became a classic, and one of the main authors, Marie Jahoda, has not been granted her one desire—she has been presented with another opportunity to study mass unemployment. And she is taking the opportunity, at Sussex University, where she now works. The Nazis did not like what she had to say about unemployment in the 1930s and burnt her book before they put her in prison. English Quakers, who knew her through her work, got her out of Hitler's prison before the war and brought her to Britain.

And it was, of course, the war that finally 'liberated' Marienthal and the rest of Europe—and the United States— from the miseries of high unemployment, only to bring new miseries. But by the time Hitler arrived in Marienthal with his soup kitchens and promise of full employment the town had experienced nine years frozen into poverty and pointlessness. One of the questions that much interested the researchers of the time, and presumably the political leaders, was whether prolonged unemployment would lead people into revolution or apathy. All the studies showed that apathy was the result.[1-3]

In Marienthal, although the local library had abolished borrowing charges, the number of readers dropped with the length of unemployment, and even those who did borrow books read fewer than before. Subscriptions to newspapers, although offered to the unemployed at a reduced price, fell by 60 per cent, and political organizations and clubs lost between one- and two-thirds of their members. Despite the flare-ups in Handsworth, Brixton, Toxteth, Southall, Moss Side, Amsterdam, Berlin, Zurich, Frankfurt, Paris, and Lille,[4,5] the picture is essentially the same today. An image that emerges time and time again from reading modern accounts of what it is like to be unemployed is of the unemployed man looking out of his kitchen window on to a completely untended garden. As Sinfield says, 'Prolonged unemployment is for most people a profoundly corrosive experience, undermining personality and atrophying work capacities.'[6]

Here then is one lesson from the 1930s that is applicable today, but I want to try to draw out others from the mass of information that accumulated at that time.[7] These lessons can seem particularly pertinent because many people who can remember unemployment in the 1930s are still alive (see box on p. 45): many of them find things worse now than then.[8] I am aware, however, of the dangers inherent in trying to draw lessons from history (the past is easily arranged to suit one's fancy), but the proximity of such a vast and dreadful 'natural experiment' makes it irresistible when many of the arguments on the effects of unemployment on health are unresolved.

More so than now unemployment in the 1930s plunged families into poverty—to the extent that 'physical deprivation in food and clothing were the rule not the exception.'[2] An average family in Britain with three children received 29s 3d unemployment benefit; food cost 20s 8d and rent 5s, which left 3s 7d for lighting, fuel, clothing, and cleaning—not enough.[2] Just as now, bigger families suffered more, and the same calculations for a family with six children resulted in a weekly deficit of 1s 11d.[2]

A working party of the Pilgrim Trust, which was chaired by the Archbishop of York and set up by him to look into the effects of unemployment, concluded that in November 1936 three out ten households of long-term unemployed men were living below a poverty line established by Mr R.F. George (partly from the British Medical Association's 'minimum standards for food requirements'); 44 per cent of these families were at or below 'a bare subsistence level.'[9] This means that they did not have enough money to keep adequately fed, warm, and clothed, and the working party describes a visit to a young couple without children in Liverpool: 'It was snow-ing outside. The house could hardly have been better kept and both of them were neatly, though not at all flashily, dressed. Yet there was no fire, and so far that day (it was 3 o'clock) they had had nothing to eat, only cups of tea . . . the man said his wife "had something for the evening" and that "they weren't starved, though sometimes they had to go pretty short. . . ." The man's statement applies to hundreds of other young couples living in such circumstances. If he had had good employment, their income would probably have been twice what it was.'[9]

The working party concluded, 'There is little doubt that many unemployed men are undernourished', and it also found that it was mothers who had the poorest diets—they made sure that their children and husbands got what there was. Other researchers found this at the time, and it still seems to be true today. Although most studies of the unemployed found evidence of malnutrition, the British government was arguing at the time that malnutrition was fast disappearing.[10, 11] Sir E. Hilton Young, the Minister of Health, said in Parliament in 1933: 'There is no available medical evidence of any general increase in physical impairment, sickness, or mortality as a result of the economic depression or unemployment.'[10] Sir John Boyd Orr, the distinguished nutritionist, in contrast, in his Chadwick lecture for 1934 estimated that there were 10 million underfed—and two years later he upped this estimate to half the population.[10]

An even starker contrast is provided by the statements of Harry Pollitt, the secretary general of the Communist Party of Great Britain, in 1933 and Sir George Newman, the retired Chief Medical Officer, in 1939.[10] Pollitt said: 'The stark reality is that in 1933, for the mass of the population, Britain is a hungry Britain, badly fed, clothed, and housed', whereas Newman took the view: 'English people, on the whole, are today better fed, better clothed, better housed and better educated than at any time of which we have record; and they enjoy a larger life and opportunity than ever before.' (The reference to English rather than British people is important because health was much worse in Scotland: infant mortality was a third higher.) Webster, who is my source for both of these quotes, has analysed the reasons for the gaps between the official and other views and concluded that the official data on nutrition are based on totally unsound foundations. Other contemporary historians take a different

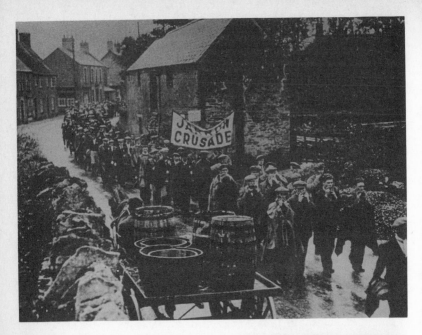

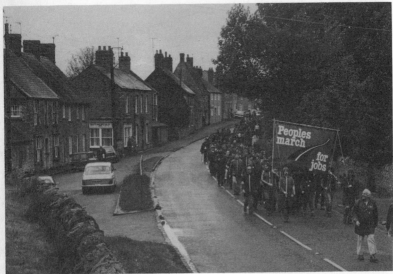

PLATE 3.1 The Jarrow Crusade, 1936 (top), and the People's March for Jobs, 1981, (below), at the same spot in Lavenden, Bucks (photograph and copyright Martin Jenkinson).

view, and one has suggested that 'child health improvements in the face of interwar depression sheds some doubt on totally pessimistic accounts of living conditions.'[12] Thus the divisions of the 1930s continue today.

Something else that has contemporary echoes was the restricting of benefits. Fear of the means test of the 1930s still goes very deep in the labour movement and is one of the causes of strong left-wing support for universal benefits. Webster describes the bureaucracy that came to surround giving free milk to mothers and young children: 'Besides completing six separate forms, applicants were subjected to an inspection by a health visitor; recent pay tickets of husbands and birth certificates were examined; and corroborating information was sought from pensions offices and public assistance authority. . . . Applicants were submitted first to a means test and then to a medical test to confirm that milk was "essential on grounds of health" in accordance with the procedure outlined in circular 185 (1921). Even if milk was granted each case would be reviewed each month.'[10]

Just as today, the psychological health of the unemployed was more studied than their physical health, but none of the studies from

---

(1) Man, single, aged 40. In normal health until unemployed. After four years' unemployment complained of choking and pains in the head, but specialist reported no lesion. Later developed alleged throat trouble, but again specialist found no physical signs. Finally, had severe stomach pains for which there was no organic explanation. Only psychological explanation adequate.

(2) Man, married (with family), aged 50. In normal health until unemployed. Developed constant aches and pains in head and became a chronic neurasthenic.

(3) Man, single, aged 22. Normal health until unemployed. Began to suffer from 'vague fears' after period of unemployment. Was admitted to hospital. Neurosis diagnosed.

(4) Man, aged 39. Normal health until unemployed. Complained of severe abdominal pains for which X-ray examination revealed no cause. Later developed other signs of neurasthenia.

Cases quoted by Dr J.L. Halliday in an investigation carried out in Glasgow and published in the *British Medical Journal* [Halliday, J.L. 1935; **ii**; 85-8] the 1930s were capable of working out which came first—the poor health or the unemployment. For the vast majority of the studies did find that unemployment and poor health went together. Their other methodological weakness was they were unable to sort out how much of the poor health was related to poverty and poor housing, nutrition, and education—because even more than now the unemployed were concentrated among the poorer sections of society.

Several studies from the United States looked at physical health. Perrott *et al.* found an illness rate among unemployed families 48 per cent higher than in families with full-time workers,[13] and the United States national health survey of 1935–6 found much the same.[14] Marsh in Canada compared the health of 1000 unemployed adults with that of 1000 employed men and 270 unemployed youths by questioning and physically examining them.[15] He also reviewed the health of 600 unemployed families. The unemployed, he found, were underweight, malnourished, had poor teeth, and suffered from gastric complaints and a variety of other illnesses, including tuberculosis and venereal diseases. Half of the members and all of the children under 5 in the 600 families were malnourished.

The working party of the Pilgrim Trust, while emphasizing that 'none of us had the medical experience necessary for a thorough study', also found poor teeth, malnutrition, and a variety of physical problems.[9] It quotes the medical officer's account of four cases of men who had 'gone to pieces' after several years' unemployment (see box on p. 39), but found most problems among the wives of unemployed men. Among women there had been a 'marked increase' in anaemia, neurasthenia, septic hands, boils, and skin troubles. Anxiety, the working party thought, was at the root of the 'lowered vitality'.

The report also quotes approvingly the work of Dr Singer, who calculated that there were annually 3200 excess deaths from puerperal disease because of the depression.[16] This first ever 'time series' analysis has since been severely criticized.[17]

But undoubtedly there was a 22 per cent rise in maternal mortality from 1923 to 1933, and this gave rise to considerable political debate and spawned several reports.[11, 18] These tended either not to consider or to deny the importance of unemployment and social conditions. Sir George Newman, the Chief Medical Officer, said in 1936 that 'bad housing, slums, insanitation, domestic overcrowding, uncleanliness, and poverty' had nothing to do with maternal mortality and morbidity; the problems, he thought, were ones of personal behaviour that 'affected rich and poor alike'.[11] Privately, Webster says, Newman accepted that these factors were important but he advised the Department of Health against investing their importance because the findings would be embarassing and would demand action beyond the means of the department.

Macfarlane and Cole have looked again at the maternal mortality data and, noting the inverse relation between mortality and unemployment rates in London, have concluded that two factors were at work: poverty and inadequate care caused high rates among poor women, while easy access to risky medical interventions caused high rates among rich women.[18] Loudon has taken a wider perspective and investigated why there was no important change in maternal mortality from 1841 until the middle of the 1930s.[19] He too notes the 'reversed social class relation' and concludes that maternal mortality (unlike infant mortality) is remarkably resistant to social deprivation but remarkably sensitive to standards of obstetric care.

If maternal mortality in the 1930s was not much affected by unemployment, psychological health certainly was. The working party of the Pilgrim Trust gave considerable space to the psychological problems of the unemployed and particularly to the work of Dr J.L. Halliday, a regional medical officer from Glasgow, who looked at 1000 insured sick men to discover why they were not working. His results, published in the *British Medical Journal* of 1935,[20] showed that a third of the cases had psychoneurotic problems, and by relating the level of psychoneurosis to the length of unemployment Dr Halliday came up with a theory on the stages of unemployment: '. . . after falling out of work there is a short period of a sense of release (a holiday freedom); gradually anxiety and depression set in with loss of mental equilibrium; finally after several years, adaptation, takes place to a new and debased level of life, lacking hope as well as fear of the future.' This 'phases model' of unemployment, as it has since been called, chimed with the working party in trying to make sense of its information from the unemployed and is also discussed in the major review of the time of the psychological effects of unemployment—that of Eisenberg and Lazarsfeld.[3]

They found 112 references for their 1938 paper and wrote:

The general conclusion of practically all workers is that unemployment tends to make people more emotionally unstable . . . unemployment

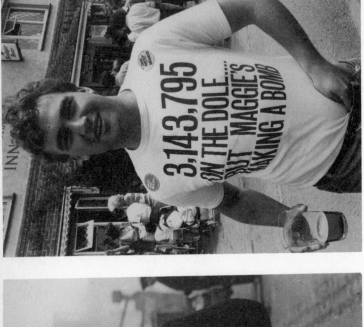

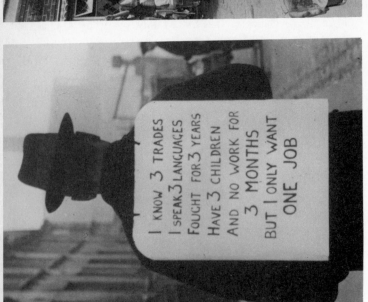

PLATE 3.2 Left: an unemployed man in the 1930s (copyright BBC Hulton Picture Library). Right: an unemployed man at the Tolpuddle rally in 1984 (photograph by Jenny Mathews, copyright Format).

represents a personal threat to an individual's economic security; fear plays a large role; the sense of proportion is shattered—that is, the individual loses his common sense of values; the individual's value is lost in his own eyes and, as he imagines, in the eyes of his fellow men. He develops feelings of inferiority, loses his self confidence, and in general loses his morale.

Eisenberg and Lazarsfeld managed to forge some sort of consensus among the various writers who had written on the phases of unemployment: 'First there is shock, which is followed by an active hunt for a job, during which the individual is still optimistic and unresigned. . . . Second, when all efforts fail, the individual becomes pessimistic, anxious, and suffers active distress; this is the most crucial state of all. And third, the individual becomes fatalistic and adapts himself to his new state but with a narrower scope. He now

---

A friend of mine has been on the idle list for the greater part of two years. This young man, a butcher's assistant, decided to give up his job in order to find something more congenial. He did so and for a time was satisfied.

But months of unemployment brought about a change of attitude. Ideals and ambitions went by the board and he would gladly have taken any situation regardless of its scope or advantages. He trudged wearily around city offices and warehouses searching for unadvertised vacancies, meeting sometimes with kindness and consideration and at other times with embarrassment and discourtesy. The mental reaction was disastrous.

Bitterness railed in his mind and he evolved strange theories regarding his inaptitude for work. In all seriousness he began to think that there was some scheme afoot to keep him unemployed. This mood of indignation invariably changed to despair. The sight of people coming to and from their places of employment became little short of a nightmare to him. Such morbid broodings led to the inevitable climax. A nervous breakdown followed which confined him to bed for several weeks. On his recovery there was a happier sequel. A job was offered him and needless to say he accepted gratefully. The work lasted six weeks and once more he was on the streets again.

Now he is a fatalist in outlook. Ambition and achievement are no longer tangible or realistic objects to his mind. Physically he is alive but mentally he is dead.

A letter quoted in *Disinherited Youth*, by the
CARNEGIE UNITED KINGDOM TRUST

has a broken attitude.' The phases model of unemployment is now rather out of favour,[21, 22] but Walter Greenwood describes the phases occurring in Harry Hardcastle in his classic novel on unemployment in the 1930s, *Love on the Dole*.[23]

The 1930s can teach us a little about responding to unemployment. War led ultimately to virtually full employment, but before that there were various attempts to reduce the misery of unemployment. In many countries free food was distributed and secondhand clothing was collected, but such endeavours could reduce only slightly the physical deprivation of unemployment. In addition, youth clubs were set up by political parties, trade unions, and voluntary organizations, but these provided neither economic independence nor a way forward.[2] In Austria a public works programme was set up in which young people were given food, clothes, and lodgings (but not wages) for a six-hour day. The scheme failed not only because it was economically inviable but also because the young saw it as a form of conscription.[2]

In 1935 in South Wales a small group of Quakers started a scheme among unemployed miners that helped 400 voluntary members produce goods and services for their own subsistence but not for wages or for sale on the open market—as the miners continued to draw their unemployment allowance.[2] The members' purchasing power was increased by about a third so that the scheme did help to compensate for the economic loss of unemployment. But could it compensate for the psychological losses? It did provide a time structure for the day and widen social contacts, and the members learnt new skills—and enjoyed working above ground. The scheme was failing, however, when the war came, particularly among the younger members, because, Jahoda thinks, it did not provide two other important commodities that paid employment brings—status and a sense of sharing the larger purpose of society. Furthermore, the miners, although they were all socialists, were worried that they were being exploited by the Quakers.

The many studies from the 1930s thus show us that the massive unemployment that affected a quarter of the workforce in Britain led to poverty with malnutrition. As a group the unemployed had more physical and psychological problems than the employed, and the rise in maternal mortality and morbidity and the slowing in the fall in infant mortality may have been related to the economic depression.

In an old fashioned parlour in a house in Sunderland, an elderly man reaches down a painted biscuit tin in which he keeps, not family photographs, but pictures of the people in Sunderland taken during the depression of the thirties. 'I take these pictures out sometimes to remind other people. I don't need reminding myself. There's not a day goes by but what I feel bitterness and shame at what this country did to millions of its working people.' The photographs, faded and cracked with age, fan out across the threadbare chenille tablecloth. He indicates a young woman with braided hair and a graceful plinth of neck. 'She came from a TB family. You knew who the TB families were, you knew not to marry into them if you wanted your children to survive. She died when she was nineteen.' There is a picture of a misty street, with a cluster of old men on the corner, hands in pockets, bodies arched against the cold. A man looks unsmilingly into the camera, flat cap, muffler parted to reveal collarless shirt. 'He was a miner. After the General Strike, he never found work again. He cut his throat one afternoon in July 1931. I can remember it like yesterday. I came home from school and found him. He'd written a message on the looking-glass with a cake of soap, saying he was sorry. He was my father.'

A council flat in the same town, October 1980. A young man with a beard, a few threads of silver in his dark hair, tries to pacify his nine month old son, while his wife, nineteen and pregnant with their third child, pushes her three year old out of the door on to the landing, and tells her not to come back until she is ready to say she's sorry. The child starts to scream, and the mother buries her face in her hands. The room is piled with washing, clothes, towels, nappies, and a few scraps of children's toys. The double bed and cot leave room for nothing but a sideboard, with a television standing on it. There is an electric kettle, a teapot, a pint of sterilised milk, a sugar bag, a sliced loaf and a tub of margarine. The young couple live with the girl's parents in their two-bedroom flat. The electricity has been cut off in their own house, the arrears of rent having reached over a hundred pounds. The husband went to London to find work, but was offered only low paid catering jobs, and could find nowhere for his family to live. He came back, even more heavily in debt, and with an even more overwhelming feeling of failure.

JEREMY SEABROOK, *Unemployment* [St Albans, Herts: Granada, 1983]

The studies of the time (and it is not so different now) were not rigorous enough to work out how much of the ill health was due to unemployment itself, how much to the unwell being more likely to become unemployed, and how much to associated factors such as poverty and poor housing. But the historical evidence shows clearly that the government tended to play down or even ignore much of the evidence associating poor health with unemployment. It was also unwilling to accept what has now become established beyond question in academic circles, although it has been questioned by members of the present government, that mortality varies greatly with social class. Another lesson is that attempts to provide the benefits of work through other institutions did not work well.

We must remember that there are considerable differences between now and 1930. Firstly, although there is extensive and increasing poverty in Britain, physical deprivation is not as extreme now. This might mean that the effects of unemployment on physical health could be lessened, but the effects on psychological health could be either lessened or increased. A second change, as Jahoda has said, is that the modern unemployed have spent more time in school (which does not necessarily mean that they are better educated).[24] Again this might reduce the harm done to psychological health because people will have more resources to cope or, alternatively, increase the harm because their aspirations might be greater and so their unhappiness with their limited lot more severe. Jahoda also thinks that the decline of the Protestant work ethic, which held that hard work would bring salvation in the hereafter, may mean that people are less concerned about being unemployed. I see little evidence for this—most surveys show that the unemployed want a job more than anything.

After his travels among the unemployed, during which he particularly sought out those who knew unemployment in the 1930s, Seabrook reached the melancholy conclusion that unemployment now is probably more damaging than in the 1930s.[8] He does not dispute that material conditions have improved, but the destruction of working class communities and traditions together with the redundancy of many of their skills means that the working class unemployed are much more lost and alone than in the 1930s. This is particularly conspicuous among the young unemployed: 'They have been nurtured in a closed world of material things brought to perfection,

We will conclude with verses written by one of the young married men, aged 23, a general labourer with almost four years of unemployment in the first seven of his industrial life.

Unemployed

I can see them standing waiting,
In the cold and drenching rain.
I can see their white drawn faces
Smiling through their grief and pain.
I can see their paltry earnings,
As they draw them from the dole.
And the thought of such corruption
Kindles anger in my soul.

Do those men whom fortune favours
And whose lives are well enjoyed,
Never think of starving brothers
In those crowds of unemployed?
Some will say they are not worthy
Of the right to draw relief,
But within their heart's deep cavern
It is not their true belief.

We are all one common people
Bound from birth on earth to dwell,
Taught to aid the sick and suffering
Not to crush their souls in hell.
But to-day the suffering lingers,
Helping hands are still and void,
And we see increasing numbers
In the ranks of unemployed.

Have we just to stand and watch them
Coming to and from the dole,
While the seething pangs of hunger
Eat into their very soul.
Can't we give a decent living,
Don't we see that dangers lurk.
If we hide the world's abundance
From those people out of work.
Then let's unite in mass formation
Human sufferings ne'er avoid,
Let's remember we have brothers
In those crowds of unemployed.

R.H.

From *Disinherited Youth*, by the CARNEGIE UNITED KINGDOM TRUST goods that cry their competitive desirability at them from the moment they are born. Their only business, its seems, is to yearn and strive for possession of them. . . . Nothing is demanded of the young but their continued passivity and quiescence. Nothing is asked of them. They seem to have no place in the world, except as obedient and abject competitors for all that is tantalisingly held out to them.'

There is, too, the terrible feeling that unemployment may be for ever. And who can forget that it was world war that got rid of unemployment last time and the time before? The next world war may sweep away unemployment for ever.

References

1. Jahoda, M., Lazarsfield, P.F., Zeisl, H. *Marienthal: the sociography of an unemployed community*. London: Tavistock Publications, 1972. (German edition published 1933.)

2. Jahoda, M. *Employment and unemployment*. Cambridge: Cambridge University Press, 1982.

3. Eisenberg, P., Lazarsfeld, P.F. The psychological effects of unemployment. *Psychol. Bull.* 1938; **35**: 358-90.

4. Lord Scarman. *The Brixton disorders 10-12 April 1981*. London: HMSO, 1981 (Cmnd 8427).

5. Williams, S. *A job to live: the impact of tomorrow's technology on work and society*. Harmondsworth: Penguin, 1985.

6. Sinfield, A. *What unemployment means*. Oxford: Martin Robertson, 1981.

7. Janlert, U., Dahlgren, G. *Unemployment, health, and the labour market— some aspects of public health policy*. Stockholm: Swedish Government, 1983.

8. Seabrook, J. *Unemployment*. St Albans, Herts: Granada, 1983.

9. Pilgrim Trust. *Men without work*. Cambridge: Cambridge University Press, 1938.

10. Webster, C. Health, welfare, and unemployment during the depression. *Past and Present* 1985; No. 109 (Nov.): 204-30.

11. Webster, C. Healthy or hungry thirties? *History Workshop J.* 1982; **13**: 110-29.

12. Holton, B. The interwar depression and social welfare on Clydeside with particular reference to the work of the education authorities. (Unpublished paper.) Quoted in: Webster, C. Healthy or hungry thirties? *History Workshop J.* 1982; **13**: 110-29.

13. Perrott, G. St J., Collins, S.D. *Sickness and the economic depression.* Washington: US Public Health Service, 1933. (US Public Health Reports 41.)

14. The National Health Survey 1935-6. *Illness and medical care in relation to economic status.* Washington: US Public Health Service, 1938.

15. Marsh, L.C. *Health and unemployment.* Oxford: Oxford University Press, 1938.

16. Singer, H. *Unemployment and health.* Pilgrim Trust Unemployment Inquiry interim paper. London: Pilgrim Trust, 1937.

17. Stern, J. *Unemployment and its impact on morbidity and mortality.* London: London School of Economics Centre for Labour Economics, 1981.

18. Macfarlane, A., Cole, T. From depression to recession—evidence about the effects of unemployment on mothers' and babies' health 1930s-1980s. In: Durward, L., ed. *Born unequal: perspectives on pregnancy and childrearing in unemployed families.* London: Maternity Alliance, 1985.

19. Loudon, I. Obstetric care, social class, and maternal mortality. *Br. Med. J.* 1986; 606-8.

20. Halliday, J.L. Psychoneurosis as a cause of incapacity among insured persons: a preliminary inquiry. *Br. Med. J.* 1935; ii: 85-8.

21. Sinfield, A. *What unemployment means.* Oxford: Martin Robertson, 1981.

22. Warr, P. Twelve questions about unemployment and health. In: Roberts, R., Finnegan, R., Gallie, D., eds. *New approaches to economic life.* Manchester: Manchester University Press, 1985.

23. Greenwood, W. *Love on the dole.* Harmondsworth: Penguin, 1969. (First published 1933.)

24. Jahoda, M. The impact of unemployment in the 1930s and the 1970s. *Bulletin of the British Psychological Society* 1979; **32**: 309-14.

4

'Gissa job'
The experience of unemployment

OTHER than losing your job (not voluntarily quitting it) and taking a long time to get another one, the best way to begin to understand the 'truth' about unemployment and to get within the skin of the experience is probably not to read reviews in the *Journal of Applied Psychology* or the *British Medical Journal* but to go and 'hang around' on street corners in Sunderland, Wigan, or Brixton. There is, of course, a strong tradition of this sort of approach—Orwell[1] did it in the 1930s and Campbell[2] and Seabrook[3] have done it in the 1980s. Indeed, in the 1930s the gap between academic and literary/political/observational studies (call them what you will) was not as wide as it is now, and the classic study by Jahoda and others on Marienthal, a one-factory town in Austria where almost everybody was unemployed for nine years, grew from her and her politically committed friends leaving the lusher pastures of nearby Vienna and going to see what they could do to help the unemployed of Marienthal.[4] They were 'scientists' who did not believe in fading into the background.

In a similar vein, the outstanding review of all the work done in the 1930s on the psychological effects of unemployment places great importance on the writings of those with inside experience: it starts by imploring its scientific readers to try to grasp the 'full, poignant, emotional feeling' of unemployment by reading a selected list of 'novels, plays, and case material'.[5] Novels take longer to incubate than journalism so we must wait for the best of the novels on unemployment in the 1980s, but in addition to the writings of Campbell and Seabrook and a host of rather dry studies of unemployment we have had Alan Bleasdale's popular television series, *The Boys from the Blackstuff*, Fagin and Little's descriptions of unemployment in families,[6] Marsden's verbatim accounts from the unemployed (accompanied by Duff's photographs),[7] and a series in the *British Medical Journal* of the experiences of general practitioners in dealing with unemployed people in their practices.[8-15]

Anybody who concentrates mostly on the more statistical and scientific studies needs often, I think, to return to these first-hand accounts of what it is like to be jobless. Studies of the associations between unemployment and various measures of physical and psychological health are beset by methodological problems, and those who are more interested in statistics than individuals may begin to feel that the damage done to health by unemployment has been exaggerated. It is then that you must go back to the accounts because they paint a desperate and painful picture. Most people who are jobless for any length of time hate the experience and long for a job: their lives, experiences, and relationships begin to empty and count for much less. Harrison described it well when he said 'Prolonged unemployment is for most people a profoundly corrosive experience, undermining personality and atrophying work capacities.'[16] Worse still, many of the long-term unemployed are ashamed, horribly ashamed (see box).[1, 3, 17]

To help readers return to these first-hand accounts I intend to include throughout this book some of the voices of the unemployed. The pictures will also, I hope, help those who have never experienced prolonged unemployment to understand more of what it is like. In the rest of this chapter I want to give some information on how much money the unemployed have, what they do, what they eat, and how they live. This sounds as if I am about to describe a race apart, and perhaps for the long-term unemployed that is not inaccurate, but the unemployed are not a uniform group—many of them will find a job within weeks or months of leaving their last one.[18, 19]

> When I first saw unemployed men at close quarters, the thing that horrified and amazed me was to find that many of them were *ashamed* of being unemployed. . . . At the time nobody cared to admit that unemployment was inevitable, because this meant admitting that it would probably continue. The middle classes were still talking about 'lazy idle loafers on the dole', and saying that 'These men could all find work if they wanted to', and naturally these opinions percolated to the working men themselves.
>
> GEORGE ORWELL *The Road to*
> [London: Victor Go

The long-term unemployed are likely to slip into poverty. The Department of Health and Social Security's cohort study of 2300 men who became unemployed in the autumn of 1978 showed that nearly half were receiving benefits worth less than half of their former take home pay,[20] and another DHSS study of those who had been unemployed for more than a year showed that 60 per cent had an income less than half of what it had been when they were in work.[21] One effect of this fall in income is that many people cannot pay their mortgages. The number of people six to twelve months in arrears with their payments tripled between 1980 and 1984 (from 13 490 to 41 900) and the number of repossessions increased from 3020 to 10 950.[21a] The National Consumer Council estimates that unemployment accounts for about 40 per cent of the arrears.[21a]

The benefits to which the unemployed are entitled include unemployment benefit and supplementary benefit. Many of the unemployed do not receive unemployment benefit, either because they have not fulfilled the contribution conditions or because they have been unemployed for more than a year. Because many do not receive unemployment benefit, because it has been cut in recent years, and because the earnings-related supplement has been abolished, an increasing proportion of the unemployed have come to depend on supplementary benefit: 52 per cent in 1980–81 but 71 per cent in 1984–5.[22] Unlike employment benefit, supplementary benefit is means tested and extra money is paid for children. Problems with supplementary benefit include some people not taking it up, difficulties for married women in claiming it, and the fact that the higher long-term rate is not paid to those who have been unemployed for over a year. The unemployed are the only group not eligible for the higher rate that is paid to all other categories of claimants who have been claiming for a year or longer.

There is no official poverty line, but many researchers take the amount available on supplementary benefit as the line. How much should be available to those living on supplementary benefit is a very political issue. Those on the right believe that it should provide for the barest necessities—food, shelter, clothing—and no more. Sir Keith Joseph (until recently a member of the Cabinet) and Jonathan Sumption argued in 1979 that a 'a family is poor if it cannot eat.'[23] And as they observed people receiving supplementary benefit riding on buses and watching television they concluded that the benefit was set too high. Most researchers, however, take the opposite view: Townsend, author of the biggest study on poverty in recent years, concluded that poverty begins when income drops below 140 per cent of supplementary benefit.[24]

The government says that supplementary benefit 'is intended to cover food, fuel, the purchase, cleaning, and repair of clothing and footwear, normal travel costs, laundry, general household expenses, and leisure and amenity items'.[25] The government's advisory committee on social security has said that it should enable recipients 'to participate in the life of the community'. This means that they should be well fed and well enough dressed to maintain self-respect and attend job interviews with confidence, have a warm home, be able to give presents to children at birthdays and Christmas, and be able to afford a newspaper and a television.[26]

Most of the evidence suggests that supplementary benefit does not provide these essentials to many claimants. In an official survey carried out in 1974 only one in 20 of the unemployed on supplementary benefit said that they were coping well—and most of those were single men.[27] Three-quarters of the men with children did not have one complete change of clothing, a warm coat, and two pairs of shoes. A more recent study looked at 1800 claimants and found that one-third of the children did not have a warm coat and half had only one pair of shoes.[28] Among parents 60 per cent lacked a standard item of clothing (a warm coat or a change of shoes), and half of the couples with children ran out of money before each week was up. Berthoud, the author, concluded: 'To run out of money more than occasionally is a pretty miserable life. To run out most weeks must make a lot of people near to desperation. Yet 38 per cent of non-pensioners and 51 per cent of couples with children reported that near desperate situation and many others were not far from it.'[28]

Campbell has described what these statistics mean in human terms: 'One man and woman in their early 20s living in Coventry with one child, mostly unemployed since leaving school, have a total income of £63 (prices are for 1982–3), including £5.25 child benefit. Weekly bills total £46.36 (rent £27.36, loan payment £3, sheets and blanket club £5, television hire purchase £2, electricity £4, gas £3, and bike payments £2) and their average diet is toast and porridge for breakfast, nothing at mid-day (the child has school dinners), sandwiches or beans on toast at tea time, cooked meals only at weekends, usually sausages or chicken and vegetables. Sometimes the woman gets vegetables from her father's garden. This is what she spent on her last three pairs of shoes: £3.99 in 1977, £9 in 1980 (when she was working) and £4.99 in 1982. She has never possessed boots or winter shoes: "I can't afford closed-in shoes, so I always wear sandals and in the winter I just put on two pairs of socks." She never buys a paper and never goes out for the evening.'[2]

Most of the recent concern over diet in Britain has been about people eating too much, particularly too much animal fat, and, although the Black report suggested that some children were under-nourished,[29] studies on undernutrition rather went out of fashion. Now as poverty is expanding such studies are reappearing. *Jam Tomorrow* was one of the first and was carried out in Manchester at the end of 1983 and beginning of 1984. The group surveyed the diets of 1000 people on low incomes (about two-thirds had an income less than £50 a week) in the north of England; 154 of these were unemployed.[30]

More than a third of the unemployed said that they or their families had had to go without a meal in the last year because they did not have enough money to buy food, and a quarter said that they did not have enough money for food all week. More than a third (39 per cent) said that when short of cash they cut back on food, and a fifth did not have a main meal every day because of the cost; half did not have three meals a day. The whole group were asked what they ate when short of money: 38 per cent said toast or bread, 34 per cent eggs, 33 per cent beans, and 32 per cent chips. More than a third (36 per cent) had eaten chips in the previous 24 hours, and 56 per cent said that they ate them several times a week or every day. In contrast, 20 per cent said that they hardly ever or never ate fresh meat and 15 per cent rarely or never had fresh or frozen fruit or vegetables.

This survey was not formally controlled but 51 people with family incomes above £150 answered the survey and gave very different answers: none had gone without a meal in the last year because of lack of money: though one said that she did not have enough money for food all week; and, although six said that they cut back on food when short of money, 24 said that they cut back on holidays. The unemployed also showed more signs of hardship than the other groups with low incomes.

The report includes some examples of the diets of the unemployed: one 25-year-old woman with a 12-month-old baby had four cups of coffee with milk but nothing else during the day and then one tin of soup with three slices of brown bread and butter in the evening; a 37-year-old man with a wife and two children had two cups of tea with milk and sugar and two custard cream biscuits in the morning, nothing for lunch, chips, egg, peas and two slices of white bread and margarine in the afternoon; and then another three cups of tea and a packet of crisps before going to bed; another 42-year-old man had four slices of toast, six slices of bread and butter, and tea for breakfast, soup with three slices of bread with a biscuit and tea for lunch, and six slices of bread and margarine with tea in the evening.

The year 1986 saw two reports on diet among the poor.[31, 32] Figure 4.1 is taken from a report by the British Dietetic Association and shows how DHSS allowances do not provide enough to pay for the energy-rich diets required by children.[31] The authors found that the amount provided by supplementary benefit for food was also inadequate for the elderly, pregnant women, the mentally and physically handicapped, the mentally ill, and for some ethnic minority groups. They also found that provision was inadequate for those many people who needed special therapeutic diets—for instance, diabetics, patients with kidney disease, or those needing a low-fat diet. Young adults might thus seem to be the only group able to eat an adequate diet on supplementary benefit, but the authors also showed that these people were given insufficient to pay for the 'healthy diets' now recommended by doctors and some government committees. The cost of buying what was allowed for in government calculations was about £9.46 a week, whereas the cost of a healthy diet ranged from £9.51 to £16.30. The London Food Commission in its study found that the cost of a healthy diet was about 35 per cent more than the amount spent on food by people with low incomes.[32] It also found that the extra needs of pregnant and breastfeeding women were difficult to meet and that women were bearing the brunt of poverty by cutting back on their own food to feed their children and husbands.

People being obliged to eat an inadequate or unhealthy diet is obviously one way in which unemployment and accompanying poverty could lead to more illness and premature death. But other

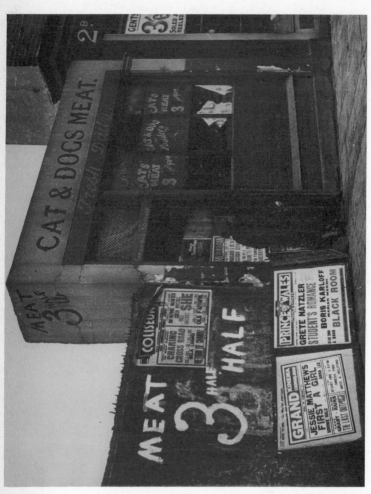

PLATE 4.1 A cat and dog meat shop near Paddington, London. Such shops were common in the 1930s and 1940s, and many poor people bought poor grade meat not for their pets but for themselves (photograph by W. Suschitzky).

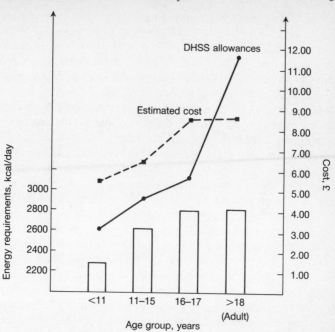

FIG. 4.1 Shows how energy requirements increase with age, and the effect this has on the cost of food.[15] For comparison the DHSS 'S' Manual guidelines for food costs are also shown. Note the considerable shortfall between the ages of 11 and 17.

changes in lifestyle—for instance, in alcohol consumption, smoking, and use of drugs—may also be important.

Some studies have suggested that the unemployed drink more alcohol than the employed and so experience more alcohol-related problems,[33-36] while some have suggested the opposite,[33, 37, 38] others have found no important relation between alcohol consumption and employment.[33, 39-41] In his general population survey of drinking Wilson found that the small group of unemployed men were more likely than employed men to be drinking above 'safe' limits.[34] The General Household Survey 1982 found that unemployed men, particularly older ones, were more likely than employed men to be heavy drinkers: among those aged 18-24, 38 per cent of the unemployed and 35 per cent of the employed were heavy drinkers;

among those aged 25–44 it was 43 per cent and 28 per cent; and among those aged 45–64 it was 25 per cent and 16 per cent.[35]

Fagin and Little, in contrast, found in their study of 22 families with an unemployed man as breadwinner that alcohol consumption fell in all but one of the families—mainly because of the expense and the decrease in socializing in pubs; one man, however, began to drink heavily, which contributed to the break-up of his marriage.[6] Alcohol consumption also fell sharply in a group of unemployed people after a steep increase in the price of alcohol in the 1981 budget in Britain.[37] The British Regional Heart Study has also produced data on alcohol consumption among the unemployed compared with the employed, and after standardization for age, social class, and town of residence the numbers of heavy drinkers among the employed and unemployed were not significantly different.[35]

These variable findings result partly from the weakness of many of the studies (most were not designed specifically to look at unemployment and alcohol consumption), partly, Crawford et al. suggest, from the different ways of measuring alcohol consumption, and partly because many different forces operate on the unemployed person.[33] Increased stress or leisure might lead him to drink more, while less money might lead him to drink less—and several studies have found a polarization in drinking habits.[33, 42, 43]

Crawford et al. looked at the drinking habits of 87 unemployed men among a population of 1503 economically active men and concluded that unemployment affects drinking styles rather than quantities consumed. The unemployed consumed the same as the employed in the week of the survey but drank faster, were more likely to have had a heavy drinking day and a binge, and suffered more consequences from their drinking.[33] However, in a longitudinal study of 44 people who lost their jobs and 26 controls Heather et al. could find no association between unemployment and changed drinking styles.[41]

Data on smoking and unemployment are less confusing—they all point to the unemployed smoking more than the employed. The General Household Survey 1982 showed that 55 per cent of the unemployed aged 16–59 were smokers compared with 38 per cent of those employed full time: the difference was considerable for both men (58 vs 38 per cent) and women (49 vs 37 per cent).[35] Fagin and Little reported an increase in cigarette consumption among both the unemployed breadwinners and their wives,[6] and Cook *et al.* found from the British Regional Heart Study more smokers among the unemployed than among the employed even after standardization for age, social class, and town of residence.[39] These cross-sectional studies do not, of course, prove that unemployment leads to more smoking.

Illicit drug use and unemployment are both very hot political issues in Britain, and many people imagine that the two are related.[44] Two British cross-sectional studies have found an association between unemployment and drug abuse.[45, 46] The British Crime Survey of 1981 showed that cannabis use among unemployed respondents was significantly higher than among other respondents.[45] An evaluation of the government's campaign against drugs showed that unemployment was one of the characteristics of the subgroup most at risk of exposure to drugs.[46] Peck and Plant[44] review other British and American studies linking unemployment and illicit drug use and note the conclusion of Catton and Shain on why people might be using heroin: 'The sense of belonging to a group, the feeling of purpose and accomplishment and the sense of prestige are all important needs which this life seems to fulfil for the user. In the conventional world these needs are much harder to satisfy for the undereducated individual who has difficulty maintaining even a menial job. The lifestyle seems to be so important that some individuals feign addiction.'[47] Sackman *et al.* have also noted that drug use may thus be fulfilling some of the social and psychological needs conventionally fulfilled by employment.[48]

My wife has known nothing but debt and poverty ever since we've been married. I know I ought to feel glad, being able to spend so much time with my kids while they're young. But what can I give them? I just feel empty. I'm ashamed I can't provide them with everything they need. What kind of a father is that? We have no life together, even though we're never apart. I've even stopped looking for work. Some days, I feel like topping myself, I'm not kidding. If there's no hope for me, what chance will they have? Life won't be worth living.

JEREMY SEABROOK A young man in October 1983 quoted in *Unemployment* [London: Quartet, 1982]

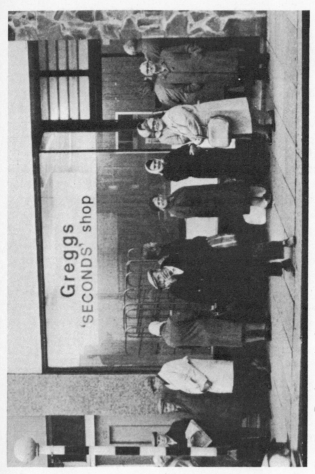

PLATE 4.2 People queueing for stale bread in Newcastle, winter 1983 (photograph by Jimmy Barnes).

The only prospective longitudinal study of unemployment and illicit drug use is that of Plant *et al.* of almost a thousand Lothian teenagers.[40, 44] They were studied first at school when 15 and 16 and then followed up: alcohol and cigarette consumption among the employed and unemployed were not significantly different four years later, but illicit drug use was significantly more common among the unemployed. Unemployed men seeking work had on average taken 1.4 illicit drugs compared with 0.5 among those in full-time employment; among those unemployed and not seeking work the figure was 2.8, hinting at an underclass. Similar differences were seen in women. Looking back at when these unemployed youngsters were at school, Plant *et al.* found no evidence that they were more 'drug oriented' than those who entered full-time employment. The melancholy reason for the unemployed youngsters not smoking or drinking more than the employed but taking more illicit drugs may be that it was cheaper to get 'out of your head' on heroin or some other illicit drug.

A further analysis found a weak but significant association between duration of unemployment and illegal drug abuse. No such association was found for alcohol or tobacco.[44] Peck and Plant also examined statistically national data on unemployment rates, addict notifications, and drug offences in Britain between 1970 and 1984 (Fig. 4.2).[44] They again found a weak but significant relation between unemployment and the two measures of illicit drug abuse.

Finally, various investigators have looked at how the unemployed spend their time. Some studies support the popular image of people getting up late, killing time, watching children's programmes on television, and taking much of the day to do something that they would have done in minutes when they were employed.[6, 49] But others do not.[50-52] Fagin and Little found in their study that the unemployed breadwinners spent more time in bed than when they had been employed but that their sleep was more restless and they felt more tired during the day.[6] The researchers also looked at the ratio of structured time (time spent doing the daily jobs that have to be done including working, and preparing and eating meals, and time spent in hobbies) to unstructured time (time spent watching the television, reading the newspaper, chatting, and 'hanging about') during unemployment and employment and were surprised to find

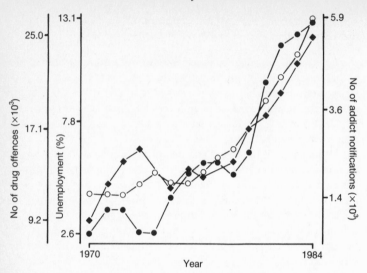

FIG. 4.2 National unemployment, addict notifications, and drug offences, 1970 to 1984: ● = unemployment; ○ = addict notifications; ■ = drug offences.

that the proportion of unstructured to structured time during unemployment increased on average 20-fold.

Miles found different results when he compared more than 300 unemployed with more than 100 employed men in the Brighton area.[50] The unemployed did not spend much more time asleep and spent only about one more hour a day in 'passive leisure', which included watching the television and listening to the radio. But they did spend three hours more a day in domestic work, including housework, shopping, and repairs, and about another hour each in 'outdoor leisure', which was mostly walking, 'mooching', and lying on the beach, and 'away from home leisure', which was mostly visiting friends and going to pubs and clubs.

Warr and Payne looked at changes in behaviour after job loss in 203 middle class and 196 working class men and found significant increases in social contact and book reading.[51] There are also significant increases in domestic work and pastimes, other pastimes, and recreations, but a significant decrease in 'entertainment through money'. Warr later confirmed these general findings in a study of 38 behaviours in 954 unemployed men.[52]

A study from Belfast that Miles quotes suggested various strategies that unemployed men adopt for filling their time: some do passively watch the television; some throw themselves into sport or religious or civic activities; some spend much time socializing; and others devote themselves to their families.[53] Despite this, most men in Miles's study said that they felt bored and restricted in what they could do—mostly because of lack of money. But one thing that unemployed men do not seem to do much is to turn to crime: Horwitz reviewed numerous studies looking for an association between unemployment and crime rates and was not able to find evidence of any strong link.[54]

References

1. Orwell, G. *The road to Wigan Pier*. London: Victor Gollancz, 1937.

2. Campbell, B. *Wigan Pier revisited*. London: Virago, 1984.

3. Seabrook, J. *Unemployment*. London: Quartet, 1982.

4. Jahoda, M., Lazarsfeld, P.F., Zeisl, H. *Marienthal: the sociography of an unemployed community*. London: Tavistock Publications, 1972. (German edition 1933.)

5. Eisenberg, P., Lazarsfeld, P.F. The psychological effects of unemployment. *Psychol. Bull.* 1938; **35**: 358-90.

6. Fagin, L., Little, M. *The forsaken families*. Harmondsworth: Penguin, 1984.

7. Marsden, D., Duff, E. *Workless: some unemployed men and their families*. Harmondsworth: Penguin, 1975.

8. Goodman, M. Unemployment in my practice: Liverpool. *Br. Med. J.* 1981; **282**: 2020-1.

9. Mackay, J. Unemployment in my practice: Govan, Glasgow. *Br. Med. J.* 1981; **282**: 2104-5.

10. Husain, M.H. Unemployment in my practice: Rotherham. *Br. Med. J.* 1981; **283**: 26-7.

11. Tanner, C.P. Unemployment in my practice: South Shields. *Br. Med. J.* 1981; **283**: 201-2.

12. Smerdon, G. Unemployment in my practice: Liskeard. *Br. Med. J.* 1981; **283**: 416.

13. Higgs, R. Unemployment in my practice: Walworth, London. *Br. Med. J.* 1981; **283**: 532.

14. Wilson, J. Unemployment in my practice: Whitehead, Carrickfergus. *Br. Med. J.* 1981; **283**: 770.

15. Jacob, A. Unemployment in my practice: Dundee. *Br. Med. J.* 1981; **283**: 1844–5.

16. Harrison, R. The demoralising experience of prolonged unemployment. *Employment Gazette* 1976; April: 330–49.

17. Greenwood, W. *Love on the dole*. London: Jonathan Cape, 1933.

18. Hawkins, K. *Unemployment*. Harmondsworth: Penguin, 1984.

19. Sinfield, A. *What unemployment means*. Oxford: Martin Robertson, 1981.

20. Moylan, S., Millar, J., Davies, R. *For richer, for poorer? DHSS cohort study of unemployed men*. London: HMSO, 1984.

21. White, M. *Long term unemployment and labour markets*. London: Policy Studies Institute, 1983.

21a. National Consumer Council. *Behind with the mortgage*. London: NCC, 1985.

22. Roll, J. Better benefits for babies—financial support for pregnancy and unemployment. In: Durward, L., ed. *Born unequal: prespectives on pregnancy and childrearing in unemployed families*. London: Maternity Alliance, 1985.

23. Joseph, K., Sumption J. *Equality*. London: John Murray, 1979.

24. Townsend, P. *Poverty in the United Kingdom*. Harmondsworth: Penguin, 1979.

25. Department of Health and Social Security. *Supplementary benefits handbook*. London: HMSO, 1983.

26. Supplementary Benefit Commission. *Annual report 1978*. London: HMSO, 1979.

27. Clark, M. The unemployed on supplementary benefit. *Journal of Social Policy* 1978; **7**: 385–410.

28. Berthoud, R. *The reform of supplementary benefit*. London: Policy Studies Institute, 1984.

29. Townsend, P., Davidson, N. *Inequalities in health*. Harmondsworth: Penguin, 1982. (Black report).

30. Lang, T., Andrews, H., Bedale, C., Hannon, E. *Jam tomorrow?* Manchester: Food Policy Unit, Manchester Polytechnic, 1984.

31. Hanes, F.A., de Looy, A.E. *Can I afford the diet?* Birmingham: British Dietetic Association, 1986.

32. Cole-Hamilton, I., Lang, T. *Tightening belts—a report on the impact of poverty on food*. London: London Food Commission, 1986.

33. Crawford, A., Plant, M.A., Kreitman, N., Latchman, R.W. Unemployment and drinking behaviour: some data from a general population survey of alcohol use. *Br. J. Addict.* (in press).

34. Wilson, P. *Drinking in England and Wales.* London: HMSO, 1980.

35. Office of Population Censuses and Surveys. *General Household Survey 1982.* London: HMSO, 1984.

36. Cobb, S., Kasl, S.V. *Termination: the consequences of job loss.* Washington DC: National Institute for Occupational Safety and Health, 1977.

37. Kendell, R.E., Roumanie, M. de, Ritson, E.B. Influence of an increase in excise duty on alcohol consumption and its adverse effects. *Br. Med. J.* 1983; **287**: 809–11.

38. Plant, M.A. *Drinking careers: occupations, drinking habits, and drinking problems.* London: Tavistock, 1979.

39. Cook, D.G., Cummins, R.O., Bartley, M.J., Shaper, A.G. Health of unemployed middle aged men in Great Britain. *Lancet* 1982; **i**: 1290–4.

40. Plant, M.A., Peck, D.F., Samuel, E. *Alcohol, drugs, and school leavers.* London: Tavistock, 1986.

41. Heather, N., Laybourn, P., Macpherson, B. A prospective study of the effects of unemployment on drinking behaviour. *Social Psychiatry*, in press.

42. Regional Working Party on Problem Drinking. *Drinking problems in North East England.* Newcastle upon Tyne: North East Council on Alcoholism, 1983.

43. Yates, F., Hebblethwaite, T., Thorley, A. *Drinking in two North East towns: a survey of the natural setting for prevention.* Newcastle upon Tyne: Centre for Alcohol and Drug Studies, 1984.

44. Peck, D.F., Plant, M.A. Unemployment and illegal drug use: concordant evidence from a prospective study and national trends. *Br. Med. J.* 1986; **293**: 929–32.

45. Mott, H.J. Self-reported cannabis use in Great Britain in 1981. *Br. J. Addict.* 1985; **80**: 37–43.

46. Research International. *Heroin misuse evaluation campaign.* London: Research Bureau Ltd, 1986.

47. Catton, K., Shain, M., Heroin users in the community: a review of the drug use and lifestyles of addicts and users not in treatment. *Addict. Dis.* 1976; **2**: 421–40.

48. Sackman, B.S., Sackman, M.M., de Angelis, G.G. Heroin addiction as an occupation: traditional addicts and heroin addicted polydrug users. *Int. J. Addict.* 1978; **13**: 427–41.

49. Jahoda, M. *Employment and unemployment: a social psychological analysis*. Cambridge: Cambridge University Press, 1982.

50. Miles, I. *Work, wellbeing and unemployment: a study of men in Brighton*. Sussex: Science Policy Research Unit, 1983.

51. Warr, P., Payne, R. Social class and reported changes in behaviour after job loss. *J. Appl. Social Psychol.* 1983; **13**: 206-22.

52. Warr, P. Reported behaviour changes after job loss. *Br. J. Social Psychol.* 1984; **23**: 271-5.

53. Kilpatrick, R., Trew, K. Quoted in: Miles, I. *Work, wellbeing and unemployment: a study of men in Brighton*. Sussex: Science Policy Research Unit, 1983.

54. Horwitz, A.V. The economy and social pathology. *Ann. Rev. Sociol.* 1984; **10**: 95-119.

5

'What's the point.
I'm no use to anybody'
The psychological consequences
of unemployment

THE evidence from both the 1930s and from more recent times is strong that most people's mental health suffers when they are unemployed, although a few manage to benefit from the experience. There is no satisfactory unifying theory on why employment work is important, but Freud claimed that it ties us to reality.[1] If we are not obliged to get up in the morning and apply ourselves to a job then we are at danger of being overwhelmed by fantasy or emotion. The unemployed broken-hearted adolescent has time to dwell on her problems, while the girl working in the post office has to concentrate on her job.

Much of the evidence of the harmful effects of unemployment on mental health comes from work done in the 1930s, from individual case studies, and from literature and journalism: most spell out the destructive nature of prolonged unemployment. More recent evidence comes from descriptive studies that look at large groups of the unemployed, from 'cross-sectional studies' (where the health of unemployed people is compared with that of employed people), 'longitudinal studies' (where a group of people are followed through a time that includes some of them becoming unemployed), and 'aggregate studies' (which look at various measures—for instance, unemployment, admissions to mental hospitals, suicide, and mortality —in whole populations and then attempt to relate them using elaborate mathematical techniques).

In one recent survey of 954 men unemployed on average for five months a fifth said that their mental health had deteriorated since they lost their job.[2, 3] They reported increased anxiety, depression, insomnia, irritability, lack of confidence, listlessness, inability to concentrate, and general nervousness. Most related these changes directly to losing their jobs, but, in contrast, 8 per cent said that their psychological health had improved since becoming unemployed—almost always because they were free of the stresses of their paid jobs. Just under two-thirds of the men described their health as excellent or good, 31 per cent as fair, 8 per cent as poor, and 1 per cent as very poor. Another study of 1698 men who had been unemployed for a year produced similar results.[4] For the first study the relation between self-reported general health and length of unemployment was highly significant, and the health of those unemployed for under six months was better than that of those unemployed for over six months. The second study also found a strong correlation between self-reported health and duration of unemployment.

The next step from surveying the unemployed is to compare the health of the unemployed with that of the employed, and Warr has identified 28 of these cross-sectional studies published since 1960.[5] They show a strong association between unemployment and poor psychological health on 13 different measures (happiness, present life satisfaction, positive affect, experience of pleasure, negative affect, experience of strain, negative self-esteem, anxiety, depressed mood, psychological distress, neurotic disorder, and suicide), and the association between unemployment and poor psychological health is very strong.

What do I eat? Eggs, chips, and beans and meat only on Sundays. I never go out, never see any friends, only ever see a convener from another plant who sometimes calls me up. Sometimes I think my brain is dying. I get depressed—sometimes I shout and bawl. I'm not going mental, but I feel I might like to damage somebody. . . .

What do I do with my time? Well, there's the garden, but I'm not a gardener, I'm not going to garden for victory yet. I do nothing. I've got the tools you'd need for anything, but I never touch them. It's very difficult to get motivated. I've got a lot to do, like redoing the kitchen, but I can't.

BEATRIX CAMPBELL[21] A middle aged former machine tool engineer quoted in *Wigan Pier Revisited* [London: Virago, 1984]

The association here is with comparatively minor psychiatric illness. Only one study seems to have looked for an association between
psychosis, serious psychiatric illness, and unemployment.[6] One difficulty with doing such studies is that many people with psychotic illnesses are likely because of their illness to be unemployed or have
poor work records. In the one study that I have identified Jaco
surveyed all the new cases of psychosis in Texas in 1951–2 and compared various of their characteristics—including employment status
—with those of the whole population of the state.[6] Among 10 758
cases, 4455 (41 per cent) were not in the labour force compared with
48 per cent, the figure for the whole population, and 814 (8 per cent)
were unemployed compared with only 2 per cent of the population.
This study cannot tell us whether the psychosis led to the unemployment or vice versa. Furthermore, extrapolation from Texas in the
1950s to Britain in the 1980s would be hazardous—but this study
deserves a mention because of its uniqueness and because of the
importance of psychosis to psychiatry.

One measure of recent changes in psychological health used in
several of these cross-sectional studies is the general health questionnaire: it contains questions on lack of confidence, sleep loss through
worry, recent experience of strain, inability to concentrate, feelings
of depression, and a sense of worthlessness, and a score above 2 on
the 12-item version means that a person has a moderate chance of being
a psychiatric case. Table 5.1 shows that many more of the unemployed than the employed score above 2.[7]

TABLE 5.1. Proportions scoring above 2 on the 12-item version of the general
health questionnaire

Sample	Proportion scoring above 2
163 unemployed recent school-leavers	54
78 unemployed men	62
399 unemployed men	60
954 unemployed men	58
87 unemployed disabled people	58
985 employed recent school-leavers	20
401 employees in a relatively untroubled organization	15
103 employees in troubled organizations	25

One Australian study used both the general health questionnaire and examination by a psychiatrist to look at unemployed 16- to 24-year-olds in Canberra.[8] The questionnaire was given to 401 young people from a sample of 716 (22 per cent refused to answer, the rest either got a job or were lost for administrative reasons). Just over half (56 per cent) were thought to have a probable psychiatric disorder— two to three times the rate in the Australian community and twice that expected among Australian general practice patients of the same age. A weighted subsample of 72 was then examined by a psychiatrist, and 47 were classed as cases: one was schizophrenic, 35 were depressed, and 11 were anxious. In 20 of these patients the onset of the severe illness came after unemployment and in the absence of any other severe stress.

These results suggest that unemployment may cause a deterioration in mental health, but they do not prove the case for two reasons. Firstly, the studies do not usually control for variables such as social class, income, educational level, and housing, all of which may be associated with mental health. Secondly, those with poorer mental health might be more likely than those with better health to lose their jobs. But this problem, which arises in all research on unemployment and health, can be answered by looking at longitudinal studies.

Warr has identified eight longitudinal studies of how unemployment affects mental health.[5] They all show that unemployment leads to a deterioration in mental health and re-employment to an improvement. Warr is confident that—at least for men (the data on women are sparse)—the case has been proved that unemployment itself damages mental health.

One of the best-known longitudinal studies, which also includes cross-sectional data, was of young people in Leeds.[9] The general health questionnaire was given to 647 16-year-olds just after they left school in 1978 and to another 1096 before they left in 1979. The two groups were then followed up twice—after roughly one year, and after 18 months. The study was only of those children who had fewer than two 'O' levels (or Certificate of Secondary Education equivalents); about half of those in England who leave school each year would fall into this group.

The unemployed had a significantly higher score on the general health questionnaire (between 13.31 and 14.88) than the employed

(7.66–8.56), those in further education (8.3–9.81), or those in the Youth Opportunities Programme (7.7–9.3).

The results were also analysed by sex, ethnic group, and qualification, and, although girls tended to score higher than boys, and Asians higher than West Indians, who scored higher than whites, most of the variation in score was accounted for by employment status. The high score was likely to be seen in the unemployed regardless of sex, ethnic group, or qualifications.

The longitudinal data show that there was no significant difference in the scores at school of those who were employed at the next interview (10.61) compared with those who were unemployed (11.36). Hence there is no evidence that those who subsequently did not get jobs had poorer mental health at school. But there was a significant increase between the score at school and the score at the next interview in those who were unemployed (from 11.36 to 13.55) and a significant decrease in those who had jobs (from 10.61 to 8.41).

The general health questionnaire score of the sample as a whole was higher before the children left school than after. This may have been due to anxiety about entering the labour market at a time when recession was deepening and unemployment mounting—a hypothesis that fits with the score decreasing significantly in those who got jobs and with later evidence on the same group that scores fell sharply in the unemployed when they got jobs.[10] This hypothesis is also supported by British adolescents saying that they are more worried about unemployment than anything else, including nuclear war.[11]

Banks and Jackson are cautious enough to conclude that their results are valid only for school leavers with poor qualifications in one metropolitan area. And a later but smaller study of school leavers

---

At first it feels marvellous. It's as though you've left the rat race, you're not in it any more and you can look at it and wonder why people bother. You look at them setting off in the morning at 7.30 and coming back at night at half past five, and you think, 'Why bother?' After a bit you get bored, and by the end of the first week you're bored stiff, and you realize you haven't a place in life. You're not contributing anything: you're not doing anything to help the community along. You're a drag on everybody else really. You're a drop-out.

DENNIS MARSDEN An unemployed man quoted in *Workless*
[Harmondsworth: Penguin, 1975]

(186 males), some of whom were better qualified than those in the first study, did not find significant overall changes on the general health questionnaire score.[12] The author did, however, find a significant change in one section of the questionnaire: the unemployed suffered a loss of confidence, personal neglect, and a degree of social dysfunction. The failure to find a significant effect overall may have reflected the small size of the study, and, as Warr says, the evidence all points in the same direction, although some groups are much more harmed by unemployment than others.

One longitudinal study that started before people lost their jobs is well known because it was controlled,[13] but Cook and Shaper were fair when they described its methods as more interesting than its results.[14] The study looked at 113 men who worked in two American manufacturing plants that closed down—one in a city and the other in the country—and followed them from 4–7 weeks before the plants closed until two years afterwards; 76 controls who worked in three manufacturing plants and one university maintenance department that were not closing were also studied. All the men also kept a health diary. One of the measures recorded was the number of days out of 14 that the men 'did not feel as well as usual', which the authors called the 'days complaint score'.

The days complaint score was significantly higher for the cases in the days leading up to the closures. The scores then fell significantly by 4–7 weeks after the closures, at which time some of the men were unemployed and others had found new jobs (the authors do not give the exact proportions). By 4–8 months after the closure, when again some men remained unemployed but others had entered new jobs, the scores again rose significantly, only to fall later as most men settled into new jobs. There was no correlation with age or education.

An analysis of the scores at times when men were employed compared with when they were unemployed showed no significant difference, and Kasl et al. think that it is the changing of jobs that is more stressful than the unemployment itself. Indeed, they say that the score for men experiencing many changes (again they do not give numbers) was significantly higher than that for men experiencing few changes, which conflicts with more recent evidence. Kasl et al. may have found different results because most of their men quickly got other jobs—a quarter immediately, another half in less than two months—and the average period of unemployment was about 19 weeks. Probably both change in employment status and prolonged unemployment cause a deterioration in mental health.

Kasl *et al.* concentrated in their study on eight men who were unsuccessful in finding stable jobs and discovered that they had high scores throughout the study. This, they suggest, was evidence that poor health was interfering with their ability (or desire) to find new work rather than vice versa.

A more recent study that followed closely the methods of Kasl *et al.* produced different results: Grayson followed 310 men and women who lost their jobs when a large Canadian plant closed in December 1981.[15] The men and women were surveyed first in August 1981 and followed up until February 1984. One big contrast with the earlier study was that although 58 per cent of the employees unrealistically thought that they would find new jobs within three months, more than 60 per cent were still without work a year later. The unemployed men had a high level of stress in February 1982 and it stayed high, hardly changing at all, right through until February 1984; the pattern was similar for their wives. Again, in contrast to Kasl *et al.*, Grayson found that their health was worse than than of the employed at the time of the closure and it became steadily worse until February 1984.

Beale, a general practitioner from Calne, Wiltshire, has also found in a controlled study of the families of 80 men and 49 women who lost their jobs when a sausage factory closed in the town that consultation rates became significantly higher than in the controls from the time when the cases were told the factory was closing until two years after the closure.[16] He suggested that the threat of closure may be worse than the event itself.

Many of the descriptive studies carried out in the 1930s attempted to identify phases in the psychological changes associated with redundancy and subsequent unemployment.[17] Fagin and Little carried on this approach in their study of 22 families in whom the male breadwinner became unemployed.[18] Leonard Fagin is a psychiatrist and Martin Little a family therapist, so not surprisingly they were struck with how similar these psychological changes are to bereavement reactions.

The first stage is a shock: nobody believes that it is going to happen to him. The next phase is one of denial and optimism, 'the holiday feeling', but within a few weeks this gives way to anxiety and distress. In this stage men seek work with great energy, but repeated failures drive them into resignation and adjustment. But this is not a healthy adjustment: rather time drags, the day is empty, and the man's personality and relationships are corroded.

Sinfield, who has been studying and talking to the unemployed for more than 20 years, is not impressed by these descriptions of phases.[19] He thinks that the experience of unemployment varies enormously depending on its length and who is unemployed, and the enthusiasts for the phases model are seeing what they want to see. He is also impressed by how ignorant people are of the effects of unemployment until they lose their jobs: 'It's changed my attitude to the unemployed. I used to think they were just skivers and was quite a lot against them, but now that I've experienced it, it's no joke, man.'

The final category of studies on the effects of unemployment on mental health are 'aggregate studies', many of them by the American sociologist Harvey Brenner. In *Mental Illness and the Economy* Brenner describes finding a very high correlation between economic activity and admission rates to mental hospitals in New York State between 1841 and 1971.[20] Indeed, instabilities in the national economy are, he says, 'the single most important source of fluctuation in mental hospital admissions'. Increases in economic instability and unemployment lead to sharp increases in mental hospital admissions, and 'the single largest population which is at risk for intensive psychiatric treatment is the population whose way of life is threatened by temporary or chronic economic instability'. In those 130 years there have, of course, been enormous changes in psychiatric practice, but these have not, says Brenner, measurably affected the relation between economic instability and mental hospital admission rates. The only change is that the greater use of drugs and the growth of psychiatric treatment within the community may have meant that more people are treated under conditions of economic stress.

These aggregate studies tell us nothing about how economic instability may affect mental health, and they cannot prove that unemployment causes a deterioration in mental health. Correlation is not proof of causation, and these studies cannot separate out the effects of unemployment from the effects of poverty, housing, social conditions, and the like. Nor can we know whether increased mental hospital admissions occur among the unemployed or those still in jobs who become more vulnerable and demanding during a recession. Indeed, Brenner has warned that we may miss large effects on health by comparing the employed with the unemployed because both may be experiencing the effects.

Whether Brenner's controversial studies are right (and the consensus among those who have been studying unemployment and health for a long time seems to be that his methods are suspect even if his broad conclusions are right), the case has been made that unemployment leads to a deterioration in mental health. Now we must consider the mechanisms by which unemployment has this effect and which groups are most vulnerable. The following quote from a semi-skilled machinist who had been unemployed for two years gives many clues.

I used to get up at 6 am, like I was going to work. I thought I'd get a job in a couple of weeks, but now it's a couple of years. That's frightening, my confidence is going. When people ask me how long I've been out of work, I think, shall I lie? When you're unemployed, you feel like you've committed a crime somewhere, but nobody tells you what you've done. The first thing that happened to me was that I realized I'd become almost illiterate after years working in a factory. I fall asleep a lot, it happens if you've got nothing to do. One bloke round here, the only place he goes is to sign on the dole. Sometimes I think I'll go barmy. Of course you get depressed, you convince yourself it's you. Sometimes I feel really ashamed, especially with things like Christmas. This will be the first time I've ever not given my sisters something for Christmas.[21]

This man gives many of the reasons why unemployment harms mental health: most are to do with loss—of status, purpose, social contacts, and a time structure to the day. One of the main research thrusts now is to investigate these mechanisms. It then becomes at least a possibility that the harmful effects may be ameliorated even while high unemployment continues.

Despite this being a research growth point, it was research done in the 1930s by Marie Jahoda that has produced some of the best information.[22] She has identified important benefits that we get from employment in addition to a wage or a salary:

It imposes a time structure on the waking day; it enlarges the scope of social relations beyond the often emotionally highly charged family relations and those in the immediate neighbourhood; by virtue of the division of labour it

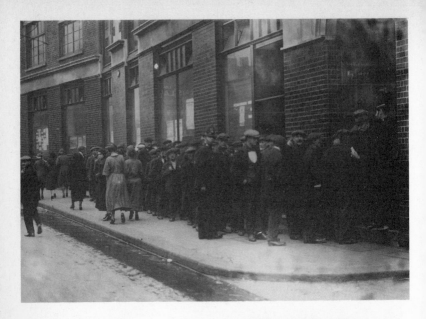

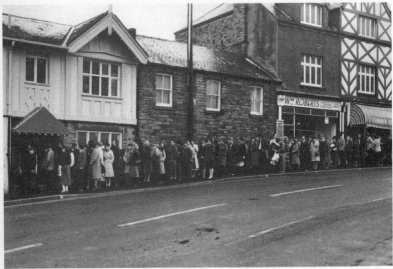

PLATE 5.1 Top: queue of unemployed people waiting outside a labour exchange in 1924 (BBC Hulton Picture Library). Below: a queue in Sheffield in February in 1983 when about 1500 people applied for 50 jobs at a restaurant (photograph by Martin Jenkinson).

demonstrates that the purposes and achievements of a collectivity transcend those for which an individual can aim; it assigns social status and clarifies personal identity; it requires regularity.

This list seems almost so acceptable as to be beyond dispute. Those of us who have a job can easily recognize that these are the benefits we get from our work, while those without one recognize what they are missing in addition to money. Of course, different jobs supply these various benefits to a greater and lesser extent, and they are to be had from other activities and institutions, but a paid job that we get up and go to most days is the main source of satisfaction for these important needs for most of us.

Miles attempted to test Jahoda's ideas in 300 unemployed and 100 employed men.[23] He asked them questions relevant to the benefits, and they kept time budget diaries and completed the general health questionnaire. The unemployed, as expected, had much worse mental health, and a complicated mathematical analysis showed that some factors related to Jahoda's benefits of work were powerful predictors of the mental health of the unemployed.

Warr has identified nine ways in which unemployment may affect psychological health,[5] and some are related to Jahoda's ideas. For Jahoda, who has lived through both of the great depressions of this century, the poverty associated with this depression is not as deep and as dreadful as that with the earlier one; but a fall in income remains important for most of the unemployed, and Warr describes it as the aspect of unemployment likely to have greatest impact on psychological health. Financial worries predict strongly overall distress scores.[24, 25]

The second factor Warr identifies is the restricted behaviours and environments of the unemployed: some do not get out and do so much or meet so many people, which is partly because they do not go to work each day and partly because they have less money.[18, 23, 26] A third problem is that the unemployed lose what psychologists call 'traction': the way that the structure of your employment pulls you along—something that you quickly achieve when you are busy and working can somehow fill your day when you have nothing in particular to do. Editors (and I am primarily an editor) understand this: when they want something done quickly they ask somebody who is busy.

A smaller scope for making decisions is a fourth problem for the unemployed person. Although he might have 'all the time in the world', he often cannot make big changes in his life because he lacks the necessary material resources. Fifthly, many of us get much of our satisfaction from developing new skills and using old ones, and mostly we do this at work. (For example, I wrote this on a word processor, which gives me considerable satisfaction despite the agonies I had at the beginning, and without work I would have had neither the money to buy the machine nor the motivation to learn to use it.)

A sixth feature is an increase in threatening and humiliating experiences: applying for jobs and being rejected; being regarded as a failure (or worse a 'scrounger'); and regular battles with unsympathetic officials at the social security office. These miseries go together with a seventh problem—feeling anxious about the future. Payne *et al.* found that a high proportion of the unemployed were anxious about the future and about becoming unemployable, losing their self-respect, and being overcome by insoluble money problems.[27]

The eighth mechanism by which unemployment harms mental health that Warr identifies is a reduced quality of interpersonal contacts[27, 28]: the woman behind the counter at the local social security office replaces the woman who came to you at work to ask for your help and your skills. This decline in the quality of interpersonal contacts is one factor that leads to the ninth and final feature, a decline in social position. Even with more than three million people unemployed, those out of work tend to think that they have failed in some way, and the status of the unemployed is low.

It got to you slowly, with the slippered stealth of an unsuspected, malignant disease. You fell into the habit of slouching, of putting your hands into your pockets and keeping them there; of glancing at people, furtively, ashamed of your secret, until you fancied that everybody eyed you with suspicion. You knew that your shabbiness betrayed you; it was apparent for all to see. You prayed for the winter evenings and the kindly darkness. Darkness, poverty's cloak. Breeches backside patched and repatched; patches on knees, on elbows. Jesus! All bloody patches. Gor' blimey!

WALTER GREENWOOD *Love on the Dole*
[Harmondsworth: Penguin, 1969 (First published 1933)]

Considerable work has also been done to work out which groups are most likely to be damaged by unemployment. One factor that is consistently found to correlate with distress is the commitment to wanting a job.[5, 29] Those who want a job most suffer most without one, and this may be one reason why a second factor, age, is important. The middle aged, who often have heavy commitments and who cannot contemplate early retirement, tend to suffer more than those who are younger or older.[30] The mental health of middle aged people also seems to deteriorate more the longer that they are unemployed, with stabilization at about six months.[31] In those who are older or younger there is no clear correlation between mental health and length of unemployment.

Beale and Nethercott warn against the common assumption that those close to the normal retiring age will not be much harmed if made redundant. The phrase 'early retirement' is well known and has desirable connotations. Beale and Nethercott excluded men over 60 and women over 55 from their main factory closure study,[16] just as others had done.[24, 32] Later, however, they analysed the consultation patterns of 10 men aged 61–64 and 10 women aged 56–59 who were laid off when the factory closed.[33] They had no controls but found a highly significant increase in both consultations and episodes of illness among the men. They consulted 66 times in the four years before closure was announced and 158 times in the four years afterwards. There was no increase among the women. Future studies should thus not ignore this group, and it may be that the men who take early retirement are a very vulnerable group.

Two other groups who suffer badly are those worst off financially and those who do the least. People in lower socioeconomic groups tend to suffer more when unemployed, which may have something to do with them having more severe financial problems.[27]

One group that seems to be protected from the psychological distress associated with unemployment is mothers in general and young mothers in particular. This may be because they have plenty of work to do, whether or not they have a job, and their responsibilities to their children provide a purpose and matter more than any other commitment.[34] But single women and women who are principal wage earners are as affected by unemployment in the same ways as men.[34]

I was in the garden again, because I didn't drink, and all I did was go in the garden. I lost meself like a bloody hermit, you know, to a large extent. I had the lads during the daytime. There was about five or six of us in the same position as meself, and we used to sit and talk, and tea-time we'd just sit there, either taking cuttings or just pottering about like a bloody old man, lost, bloody utterly. I stopped even looking for a job. In them two years I lost all bloody interest. I thought, 'What's the bloody point of it all, anyway? What's the reason for it all?' Then you start to become, well, deranged . . . I can't pronounce the word when you're thinking about things, I can't get it out . . . psychologically. You start thinking about it, 'What the bloody hell's the point? Why are you here?' I lost me interest in me religion, you know. There was a time when I thought, fair enough, there's a God and all this, that and the other, you know, but I never went to church. Now, well, I don't believe there is a God now, me. Well, anybody who thinks there's a God, he must be a funny bloody God, not my God anyway. He works the wrong way for me if there is one. I think he should look after everybody if there is one, like. I don't think there is.

> DENNIS MARSDEN An unemployed man quoted in *Workless*
> [Harmondsworth: Penguin, 1975]

One further group who suffer disproportionately from unemployment, 'the vulnerable', are those who do not cope well with any stress, and for them unemployment may be particularly painful.[5]

But, at the other end of the vulnerability scale, some people flourish when unemployed: a small minority of the unemployed feel that they have benefited from the experience.[18, 35, 36] For some the reason is simply that they have got away from a dreadful, unrewarding, poorly paid, stressful job, but others have managed to respond positively to becoming unemployed. Marsden and Duff found a man who had taken up painting after losing his job, and it had become much more important to him than his job had ever been.[35] Fagin and Little describe a man who had become equally passionate about gardening.[18] The Maternity Alliance survey of 30 young unemployed families also found that in 14 cases the fathers were grateful to have more time to be with their children.[36]

Starting from these observations, Fryer and Payne set out to find people who had responded positively to unemployment and discover how they had managed it.[37] This approach is the reverse of the traditional clinic study, which is still important in psychology, that tries to draw inferences about the normal by studying the pathological. Through community workers, Fryer and Payne found 11 people who were 'coping exceptionally well' with unemployment: six were of middle class origin, and in general they were 'upwardly mobile'—nine when employed had been I or II on the Registrar General's classification.

Fryer and Payne eschew giving individual case histories but instead lump the characteristics of the 11 together in an unsatisfactory and obscure way. But all 11 drew a distinction between work and employment: they were very interested in their work, for which they were not paid, and less interested in the paid employment that they had had in the past—although five would have liked to have had paid employment provided they could still do the work that they found fulfilling. They were very active and all had goals—usually political, religious, or personal—towards which they were striving. Most had been active throughout their lives and were good at organizing their time.

This last characteristic brings us back to Jahoda's ideas, in the light of which Fryer and Payne analysed their results. As well as imposing an internal structure to their day, all of these 11 participated in shared experience outside the home and found transcending goals and purposes outside paid employment. Thus they were finding other ways of fulfilling the needs that for most people employment satisfies.

Finally, Warr has developed ideas on 'good' and 'bad' employment and unemployment (Table 5.2) from studies on both the employed

TABLE 5.2 Characteristics of psychologically 'good' and 'bad' jobs and unemployment[38]

	Good jobs have	Bad jobs have	Good unemployment has	Bad unemployment has
Money	more	less	more	less
Variety	more	less	more	less
Goals, traction	more	less	more	less
Decision latitude	more	less	more	less
Skill use/development	more	less	more	less
Psychological threat	less	more	less	more
Security	more	less	more	less
Interpersonal contact	more	less	more	less
Valued social position	more	less	more	less

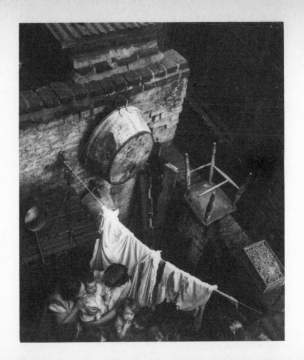

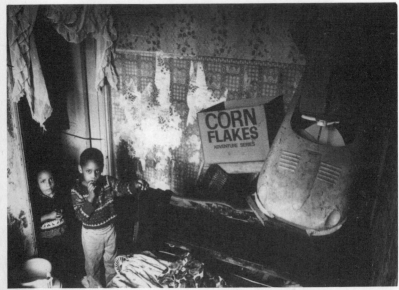

PLATE 5.2 Children looking out of poverty in the slums of the 1930s (top: photograph by Edith Tudor Hart, copyright W. Suschitzsky) and the 1970s (below: copyright BBC Hulton Picture Library).

and the unemployed, many of them done in his own unit[38]; rather like Jahoda's ideas, they have the great merit of seeming obvious. As Warr says, the priority should be to move people from bad unemployment into good employment but failing that we should aim at moving the unemployed into good unemployment.

References

1. Freud, S. *Civilisation and its discontents*. London: Hogarth, 1963.

2. Warr, P. Work, jobs and unemployment. *Bull. Br.Psychol. Soc.* 1983; **36**: 305–11.

3. Jackson, P.R., Warr, P.B. Unemployment and psychological ill health: the moderating role of duration and age. *Psychol. Med.* 1984; **14**: 605–14.

4. Colledge, M., Bartholomew, R. *A study of the long term unemployed*. London: Manpower Services Commission, 1980.

5. Warr, P. Twelve questions about unemployment and health. In: Roberts, R., Finnegan, R., Gallie, D., eds. *New approaches to economic life*. Manchester: Manchester University Press, 1985.

6. Jaco, E.G. *The social epidemiology of mental disorders*. New York: Russell Sage Foundation, 1960.

7. Warr, P. Job loss, unemployment and psychological well being. In: Allen, V.L., van de Vliert, E., eds. *Role transitions*. New York: Plenum Publishing, 1984.

8. Finlay-Jones, R., Eckhardt, B. Psychiatric disorder among the young unemployed. *Aust. N.Z. J. Psychiat.* 1981; **15**: 265–70.

9. Banks, M.H., Jackson, P.R. Unemployment and risk of minor psychiatric disorder in young people: cross sectional and longitudinal evidence. *Psychol. Med.* 1982; **12**: 789–98.

10. Jackson, P.R., Stafford, E.M., Banks, M.H., Warr, P.B. *Work involvement and employment status as influences on mental health: a test of an interactional model*. Social and Applied Psychology Unit, 404. Sheffield: University of Sheffield, 1982, (Memo 404).

11. Gillies, P., Elwood, J.M., Hawtin, P., Ledwith, F. Anxieties in adolescents about unemployment and war. *Br. Med. J.* 1985; **291**: 383–4.

12. Layton, C. Change score analyses on the GHQ and derived subscales for male school leavers with subsequent differing work status. *Personality Individ. Diff.* 1986; **7**: 419–22.

13. Kasl, S.V., Gore, S., Cobb, S. The experience of losing a job: reported

changes in health, symptoms and illness behaviour. *Psychosom. Med.* 1975; **37**: 106-21.

14. Cook, D.G., Shaper, A.G. Unemployment and health. In: Harrington, J.M., ed. *Recent advances in occupational health. Vol II.* Edinburgh: Churchill Livingstone, 1984.

15. Grayson, J.P. The closure of a factory and its impact on health. *Int. J. Health Serv.* 1985; **15**: 69-93.

16. Beale, N.R., Nethercott, S. Job loss and family morbidity—a factory closure study in general practice. *J. R. Coll. Gen. Pract.* 1985; **35**: 510-14.

17. Eisenberg, P., Lazarsfeld, P.F. The psychological effects of unemployment. *Psychol. Bull.* 1938; **35**: 358-90.

18. Fagin, L., Little, M. *The forsaken families.* Harmondsworth: Penguin, 1984.

19. Sinfield, A. *What unemployment means.* Oxford: Martin Robertson, 1981.

20. Brenner, H. *Mental illness and the economy.* Cambridge, Mass.: Harvard University Press, 1973.

21. Campbell, B. *Wigan Pier revisited.* London: Virago, 1984.

22. Jahoda, M. *Employment and unemployment.* Cambridge: Cambridge University Press, 1983.

23. Miles I. *Adaptation to unemployment.* Science Policy Research Unit memo. Sussex: University of Sussex, 1983.

24. Jackson, P.R., Warr, P.B. Unemployment and psychological ill health: the moderating role of duration and age. *Psychol. Med.* 1984; **14**: 605-14.

25. White, M. Life stress in long term unemployment. *Policy Stud.* 1985; **5**: 31-49.

26. Warr, P.B., Payne, R.L. Social class and reported changes in behaviour after job loss. *J. Appl. Social Psychol.* 1983; **13**: 206-22.

27. Payne, R.L., Warr, P.B., Hartley, J. Social class and the experience of unemployment. *Sociology Health Illness* 1984; **6**: 152-74.

28. Stokes, G. Work, unemployment, and leisure. *Leisure Stud.* 1984; **2**: 269-86.

29. Warr, P.B. A study of psychological well being. *Br. J. Psychol.* 1978; **69**: 111-21.

30. Daniel, W.W. *A national survey of the unemployed.* London: Political and Economic Planning Institute, 1974.

31. Brinkman, C. Health problems and psychosocial strains of the unemployed. In: John, J., Schwefel, D., Zollner, H., eds. *Influence of economic stability on health.* Berlin: Springer, 1983.

32. Hepworth, S.J. Moderating factors of the psychological impact of unemployment. *J. Occup. Psychol.* 1980; **53**: 139-45.

33. Beale, N., Nethercott, S. Job loss and morbidity in a group of employees nearing retirement age. *J. R. Coll. Gen. Pract. 1986;* **36**: 265-6.

34. Warr, P.B., Parry, G. Paid employment and women's psychological well being. *Psychol. Bull.* 1982; **91**: 498-516.

35. Marsden, D., Duff, E. *Workless: some unemployed men and their families.* Harmondsworth: Penguin, 1975.

36. Salfield, A., Durwald, L. 'Coping but only just'-families' experience of pregnancy and childbearing on the dole. In: Durward, L., ed. *Born unequal: perspectives on pregnancy and childbearing in unemployed families.* London: Maternity Alliance, 1985.

37. Fryer, D., Payne, R., Proactive behaviour in unemployment: findings and implications. *Leisure Stud.* 1984; **3**: 273-95.

38. Warr, P. Work, jobs, and unemployment. *Bull. Br. Psychol. Soc.* 1983; **36**: 305-11.

6

'He never got over losing his job' Death on the dole

In politics corpses matter: a few deaths may change policy in a way that an ocean of misery will not. Much energy has thus been devoted to arguing whether unemployment kills. From his aggregate studies (also known as time services analyses) Brenner has calculated that societies in which the number of unemployed increases by more than one million in five years will experience tens of thousands of excess deaths;[1-8] but Gravelle has countered under the heading 'Lies, damned lies, and time series results' by arguing that unemployment is 'not important in explaining variations in general population mortality'.[9] Scott-Samuel,[10] in his turn, has attacked Gravelle for underplaying the results of an important study based on the Office of Population Censuses and Survey's longitudinal study[11, 12] and offered his own calculation that male unemployment causes 3000 extra deaths a year in Britain.[13]

Time series analyses relate measures of economic activity and stability with measures of health in different communities over varying periods of time. Brenner is the name most associated with these studies, but Fraser attempted comparisons between different countries more than 10 years ago,[14] and Singer was using these techniques in the 1930s to try to find an association between unemployment and maternal and infant mortality and deaths from specific causes.[15]

Singer worked out differences in death rates from various causes for all the county boroughs in England and Wales from 1928 to 1933 and tried to correlate these with changes in unemployment rate. After attempting to eliminate the effects of other variables, he found statistically significant correlations between unemployment and maternal and infant mortality and deaths from diarrhoea and enteritis, diphtheria, scarlet fever, and tuberculosis. Stern, however, has recently reworked these data and found that only the correlation with maternal mortality was significant,[16] which itself conflicts with Loudon's conclusion from historical evidence that maternal mortality is remarkably insensitive to socioeconomic conditions.[17]

Morris and Titmuss tried to extend Singer's work in a paper published in 1940,[18] and Farrow has recently summarized their work.[19] They looked at deaths from rheumatic heart disease and unemployment rates in 83 county boroughs from 1927 to 1938 and found correlations between unemployment, poverty, overcrowding, and mortality. The correlation between unemployment and mortality persisted even after allowing for the correlations with poverty and overcrowding. Stern found the methods sophisticated for the time and the results persuasive but not conclusive.[16] Brenner did not know of the work of Morris and Titmuss until after he had done many of his studies and was delighted when he learnt of it. He wrote: 'These findings are nearly identical to those I have reported for the United States in all major categories of heart disease for all ages.'[1]

Computers have made aggregate analyses much easier but also more baffling: the innumerate, which by the standards of Brenner is

---

Five years ago we were a happy, contented family. My husband had a good job. I was working at North Tees Hospital. We were able to buy a nice house, we had annual holidays. If we wished to buy anything we bought it. We had a little in the bank. Then my husband fell into ill health. He was made redundant, he was 54 then and because of his age was unable to find employment. I went on to full time working at the hospital. As the years have gone on—our savings went, no more holidays, no social life at all. We began to sell our possessions. The colour TV. Our lovely grandfather clock, our rings, watches, bits of silver and brass, our stereo—anything we could sell we sold to pay the ever rising cost of living, the bills which are more each time they arrive. My son is now 15 years old, he is a big boy with a big appetite. He seems to grow overnight. It is a nightmare trying to keep up with his clothes. He is in men's clothes now, which are very expensive. He's a good boy doing very well at school and we are determined that he goes on to higher education. I have been in ill health for two years, I'm sure it is all the worry and stress of trying to cope. Both my husband and I are ex-service. Is this what we fought for?

JENNIE POPAY Extract from a letter quoted in *Unemployment and the Family* [London: Unemployment Alliance, 1984 (Unemployment Alliance Briefing Paper No. 4)]

most of us, can be bewitched by the mathematical magician. Despite computers, these studies do not allow any more confident conclusions now than they did in the 1930s and 1940s. We cannot know, for instance, whether excess deaths occur among the employed or the unemployed, and Brenner does not suggest that all the excess deaths occur in the unemployed.[2] Many, he hypothesizes, do occur among the unemployed but they probably also occur among those left in unstable work and those who lose one job and find another that is perhaps more poorly paid and more dangerous. Furthermore, the death rate tends to increase when the economy picks up again—people starting new jobs that demand new skills may experience increased mortality.

Brenner began his work by finding an inverse relation between the first admission rate to New York State mental hospitals and the employment rate from 1914 to 1967 and an index of business cycles from 1841 to 1909.[3] Next he found that for the whole of the United States homicide and suicide rates rose within a year of unemployment rising,[4] and then he moved on to looking at 'chronic physical illnesses with a stress element, especially cardiovascular diseases':[5] for most age groups and both sexes deaths from cardiovascular disease increased after a lag of two to three years. Before turning his attention to Britain, Brenner went on to relate the infant mortality rate,[6] mortality from alcohol consumption,[7] and total mortality to economic instability.[9]

In his analysis of the relation between mortality and changes in the national economy in England and Wales from 1936 to 1976, Brenner used a model with four main components: real per caput income, which shows a steady increase and is associated with improved nutrition, sanitation, and living conditions; the unemployment rate; a measure of 'rapid economic growth' derived from deviations from the steady increase in real per caput income; and government expenditure on welfare.[2] He found that long-term economic growth was negatively related and unemployment (indicating recession) positively related to mortality in all age groups. Rapid economic growth was weakly related and welfare expenditure inversely related to mortality only for those under four years old. Just as in America, deaths from suicide and homicide rose within a year, while deaths from cardiovascular disease took two to three years to increase. Brenner emphasized that the increases in mortality resulted from a slowing of the expected decline and from a widening of the long-observed differentials in death rates between different socioeconomic groups.

Later a group from London used Brenner's model over a longer time (1922 to 1976) and fed in what they argued were better data.[20] They found no statistically significant relation between unemployment and mortality. The dominant feature between 1936 and 1976 was, they pointed out, the dramatic fall in unemployment at the beginning of the war, and any analysis that included this fall was bound to find a correlation with mortality, which had been falling steeply all the time. Brenner replied by saying that he had made it quite clear that his model was applicable only to the shorter time span and could not be used in particular for years that included the 1930s depression.[21] Wagstaff has surveyed the work of both Brenner and those who have tried to replicate his model and has concluded that Brenner's analyses have not provided convincing evidence that the social costs of unemployment include premature deaths.[22] Brenner's models have, Wagstaff argues, been wrongly specified, and the unemployment variable in his calculations may well have been picking up the effects of other omitted variables. Aggregate studies have been made of Scotland by others, and these have either found no relation between mortality from all causes or a slight negative association.[23, 24]

These aggregate studies were at the centre of the debate over unemployment and health a few years ago, but their importance has now receded—partly because of their inherent limitations and partly because better studies have come along. Warr has summarized the problems with these studies.[25] Firstly, studies of correlation cannot prove causation, and, secondly, what goes for whole populations may not go for individuals within those populations. Thirdly, the authors of these studies often present few details of their findings, and when they are generating so much data and applying so many statistical tests it is easy to concentrate on the most impressive results. Fourthly, minor procedural changes—for instance, use of a different time span—produce dramatically different results. Fifthly, there are many confounding variables (those that vary with unemployment and may be the true causes of changes in health) such as changes in diet and availability of health services. Finally, these are necessarily all studies of the past and thus the results may not apply to the present—for instance, today the unemployed experience less absolute poverty than the unemployed of the 1930s, which might make a big difference in the effects of unemployment on mortality.

More important now than these aggregate studies are longitudinal studies, which follow a group of people through time as their employment status changes: these can prove causal links between unemployment and mortality. Sadly, such a specific longitudinal study was never set up in Britain—despite unemployment beginning to increase dramatically over six years ago. Clever use has been made, however, of data from the 1971 census, which did ask about employment status in the week before the census.

Moser *et al.* used data from the Office of Population Censuses and Survey's longitudinal study that follows up a 1 per cent sample of the population of England and Wales.[11, 12] They looked at 5861 men aged 15–64 (3.6 per cent of the total) who said that they were waiting to take up a job or seeking work in the week before the census. The study does not include those who were temporarily or permanently sick, retired, or otherwise inactive; nor does it include women because of the difficulty of interpreting their employment status— for instance, 38 per cent of the sample was put in the inactive category to which housewives are assigned.

The standardized mortality ratio for 1971–81 for men aged 15–64 at death who were seeking work in 1971 was 136 (95 per cent confidence intervals 122–152). It was higher in the second half of the decade (144) than in the first half (129) and was raised for all ages, although it was particularly high among those under 54, reaching over 200 in those aged 35–44 (Fig. 6.1).

Moser *et al.* calculated that some of this difference in mortality between those employed and the unemployed was due to socio-economic distribution: the mortality ratio for all unemployed men standardized for age and class was 121 (95 per cent confidence intervals 108 to 135). But within each social class the mortality was higher among the unemployed than the employed, and the difference in mortality between the highest and the lowest social classes was greater for the unemployed than for the employed. The causes of death that predominated among the unemployed were 'malignant neoplasms' (standardized mortality ratio 141), particularly lung cancer (standardized mortality ratio 175), and 'accidents, poisonings,

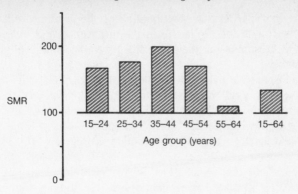

FIG. 6.1 Standardized mortality ratio from 1971 to 1981 among men seeking work in 1971, by age at death.

and violence' (standardized mortality ratio 202), particularly suicide (standardized mortality ratio 241).

Was the excess mortality among those seeking work caused by the unhealthy being more likely to become unemployed? Moser *et al.* had to be ingenious in trying to answer this question because the data had not been collected with this question in mind. They pose the hypothesis that if people were becoming unemployed because they were sick then there would be greater mortality in the whole group at the beginning of the decade compared with the end as some of these people died and the health of the group as a whole improved. In fact, the mortality before standardization for social class was higher in the second half of the decade, and after standardization there was no significant difference between the two periods.

Another method used to eliminate the 'health selection effect' is to look at the mortality of the wives of men seeking work. If unemployment itself harms health, the argument goes, then it might also harm the health of wives. The overall standardized mortality ratio for the 2906 women was 120 (95 per cent confidence intervals 102–139). Thus there seems to be an effect of unemployment on the health of wives comparable to that on their husbands. A later analysis of the mortality of women other than wives living with the men seeking work also showed a raised standardized mortality ratio of 110 (95 per cent confidence intervals 97–123).[26] The authors have also tried to explain away the excess mortality of both the men and their wives by looking at effects of marital state distribution and the combined effects of social class and housing tenure in the men and of the wives' own economic position—but they were still left with considerable excess mortality.[12]

They have also investigated whether the excess mortality among those seeking work might arise from the well-known regional differences in mortality.[26] But the standardized mortality ratios of those seeking work were raised in all three regions investigated: the North and West region (141, 95 per cent confidence intervals 118–167); the Central region (143, 95 per cent confidence intervals 116–173); and the South and East region (118, 95 per cent confidence intervals 96–143). Thus rather than explaining away the findings this analysis shows that the effect may be greater in areas with higher rates of unemployment where a man's unemployment is likely to last longer.

It must be remembered, too, that many of those who lost their jobs because they were sick would be included in the temporarily or permanently sick groups—and so would be excluded from this study. The bias is thus towards the 'healthier unemployed', but the conclusion of Moser *et al.* on whether unemployment *per se* causes increased deaths is suitably restrained: 'Although these data provide no strong evidence for a selection effect, we cannot rule out the possibility that there is one operating. The complexity of the hypothesis and the large sampling variation make conclusive interpretation of the data difficult.' But we should not, I think, become too obsessed with trying to work out whether poor health or unemployment comes first because either way it adds up to a great many people in poor health not having jobs.

Another problem with concluding too much from this study is that unemployment was about 4 per cent in 1971 but is now over 13 per cent. As unemployment has grown so the characteristics of the unemployed have changed; unemployment is now much commoner among the middle aged and the middle class, in whom it was rare in times of fuller employment. Possibly any effect whereby the unhealthy are more likely to lose their jobs may operate more strongly when fewer people are unemployed. The researchers thus warned against extrapolating from their findings to estimate the impact of unemployment on health today.

But they have now had a chance to begin to analyse the data from the 1981 census.[27] In this sample the number of men in employment fell from 87 to 81 per cent, but as well as the number of men seeking work increasing there was also a considerable increase in the number reporting themselves retired or permanently sick. These groups, which have high standardized mortality ratios, are likely to include some unhappy men who have been forced into premature retirement or who have opted for the reduced stigma, and better benefits, of the sick compared with the unemployed.

A comparison of the data for 1971-3 and those for 1981-3 shows a very similar pattern. The standardized mortality ratio for 1971-3 of men seeking work was 121 (95 per cent confidence interval 98-147) and for 1981-3 it was 112 (95 per cent confidence interval 96-129). The other analyses done on the 1971 data also produce similar results when repeated on the 1981 data. If these findings are confirmed after long follow-up they will add greatly to the evidence showing that unemployment kills.

Despite the author's warnings against extrapolating from the earlier data, Scott-Samuel has been unable to resist making a few calculations. He calculates that if the population-attributable risk of death associated with unemployment has remained constant and if the risk applies equally to the whole of Britain then the number of deaths from male unemployment in 1984 in Britain would have been 2125 among men and 1077 among their wives.[13]

Some other data that give a little more insight into whether unemployment kills comes from a New York study of 2320 men who had survived a heart attack and who were then entered into a therapeutic trial.[28] The researchers conducted psychosocial interviews with all these men at the beginning of the trial and then assigned them to high or low levels of life stress and social isolation. A man was rated as having high life stress if he said that he was retired but would prefer to be working. Social isolation was not related by the authors to unemployment. Three-year follow up showed that even when other important prognostic factors were controlled for, the risk of death was four times higher in the men who had high levels of life stress and who were socially isolated compared with those who had low levels of stress and who were not isolated.

Not too much can be concluded about unemployment and mortality from this study as these were men who were already unwell with one particular condition and unemployment was only one of many factors considered. But it does illustrate how doctors in their everyday working lives should be paying attention to factors like unemployment.

It has not been proved that unemployment kills, but the circumstantial evidence is strong and many studies point in the same direction. But those who want proof as strong as the proof that cigarette smoking causes lung cancer will probably never have it. This is as much a reflection of the difficulty of the problem—with its many confounding variables—as of the inadequacies of the studies. Also, any association that there may be between unemployment and death cannot be nearly as strong as that between smoking and death.

As there is no consensus that unemployment leads to an increase in mortality, not surprisingly there has been little research into mechanisms; nevertheless, when thinking about unemployment and health, there is a tendency, which has to be resisted, to adopt sooner or later an oversimplified model: changes in the economy are seen as the cause of the problem of unemployment, which leads in turn to the result of poor health and death. Spruit has criticized this model,[29] and Svensson has proposed a more complex one.[30] But the best model so far comes from the Unemployment and Health Study Group (Fig. 6.2).

We must not dismiss as an epidemiological nuisance the complicating factor that the unhealthy are more likely than the healthy to find themselves without a job. Some of these sick people will feature in the unemployed statistics and so lead to an association between unemployment and premature death; but others will be classified as long-term sick or prematurely retired and so will not contribute. Furthermore, double jeopardy operates: those who lose their jobs because they are unhealthy, a vulnerable and ailing group, are then subjected to the full misery of unemployment and a further deterioration in health. Many of these people are unskilled middle aged men, some of them probably heavy smokers and drinkers, who are ripe for developing heart disease.

So how might unemployment cause death? The proved deterioration in mental health associated with unemployment may cause death not only through suicide but also through aggravating physical illnesses and reducing people's ability and will to recover from them. Epidemiologists have made little progress with sorting out the importance of mental health in conditions such as heart disease,[31] and they are always tempted to ignore it because of 'measurement problems'. But even measuring blood pressure can be difficult, and the talk of 'measure-

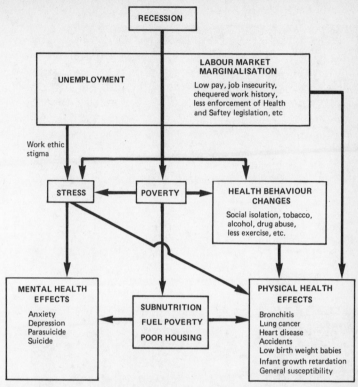

FIG. 6.2 How might unemployment lead to poor health? [Unemployment and Health Study Group, 1986]

ment problems' may hide an ingrained or inbuilt impatience with trying to sort out how an ailing psyche may lead to physical disease, which may mean that substantial effects of unemployment on physical health and mortality are not being elucidated.

Poverty is the next way in which unemployment may lead to poor physical health—because unemployment leads to poverty and poverty leads to poorer health and higher mortality.[32, 33] It does this in a myriad of unelucidated ways, but poorer living conditions and reduced access to medical services are among the most important.

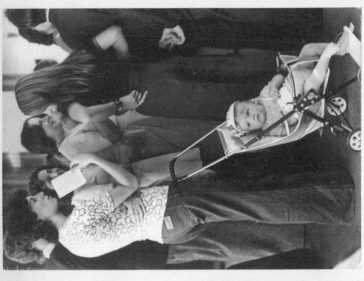

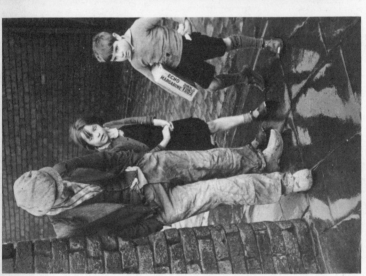

PLATE 6.1 Left: unemployed man in Wigan 1939 (BBC Hulton Picture Library). Right: women queueing for work in Kirkby employment exchange 1975 (picture by John Sturrock, copyright Report).

The inadequate diet of the unemployed must harm health, but so may changes in tobacco and alcohol consumption, drug taking, and general lifestyle. The harm caused by some of these factors may not become apparent for many years.

Finally, much of the damage associated with unemployment may be experienced not only by those without any job but also by those who worry about losing a job, accept poorer working conditions rather than leave a job, leave relatively good jobs to pass through a series of poorly paid and perhaps dangerous jobs, put together an inadequate and insecure living in the black economy, or are pushed against their will into premature retirement. These groups constitute the non-employed or the sub-employed, and researchers are increasingly focusing on them.[34]

References

1. Brenner, M.H. Unemployment, economic growth, and mortality. *Lancet* 1979; **i**: 672.

2. Brenner, M.H. Mortality and the national economy. *Lancet* 1979; **ii**: 568–73.

3. Brenner, M.H. *Mental illness and the economy*. Cambridge, Mass.: Harvard University Press, 1973.

4. Brenner, M.H. *Time series analyses of relationships between selected economic and social indicators*. Springfield, Virginia: United States National Technical Information Service, 1971.

5. Brenner, M.H. Economic changes and heart disease mortality. *Am. J. Pub. Health* 1971; **61**: 606–11.

6. Brenner, M.H. Fetal, infant, and maternal mortality during periods of economic instability. *Int. J. Health Serv.* 1973; **3**: 145–59.

7. Brenner, M.H. Trends in alcohol consumption and associated illnesses: some effects of economic changes. *Am. J. Pub. Health* 1975; **65**: 1279–92.

8. Brenner, M.H. Health costs and benefits of economic policy. *Int. J. Health Serv.* 1977; **7**; 581–623.

9. Gravelle, H. *Does unemployment kill?* London: Nuffield Provincial Hospitals Trust, 1985.

10. Scott-Samuel, A. Does unemployment kill? *Br. Med. J.* 1985; **290**: 1905.

11. Moser, K.A., Fox, A.J., Jones, D.R. Unemployment and mortality in the OPCS longitudinal study. *Lancet* 1984; **ii**: 1324–9.

12. Moser, K.A., Fox, A.J., Jones, D.R., Goldblatt, P.O. *Further analyses of unemployment and mortality in the OPCS longitudinal study.* London: Social Statistics Research Unit, City University, 1985.

13. Scott-Samuel, A. Unemployment and health. *Lancet* 1984; **ii**: 1464–5.

14. Fraser, R.D. *Int. J. Health Serv.* 1973; **3**: 3.

15. Singer, H. *Unemployment and health.* Pilgrim Trust Unemployment Enquiry Interim Paper. London: Pilgrim Trust, 1937.

16. Stern, J. *Unemployment and its impact on morbidity and mortality.* London: London School of Economics Centre for Labour Economics, 1981.

17. Loudon, I. Obstetric care, social class, and maternal mortality. *Br. Med. J.* 1986; **293**: 606–8.

18. Morris, J.N., Titmuss, R.M. *The Medical Officer* 1940; **2**: 69.

19. Farrow, S.C. Monitoring the health effects of unemployment. *J. R. Coll. Physicians Lond.* 1983; **17**: 99–105.

20. Gravelle, H.S.E., Hutchinson, G., Stern, J. Mortality and unemployment: a critique of Brenner's time series analysis. *Lancet* 1981; **ii**: 675–9.

21. Brenner, M.H. Unemployment and health. *Lancet* 1981; **ii**: 874–5.

22. Wagstaff, A. Time series analysis of the relationship between unemployment and mortality: a survey of econometric critiques and replication of Brenner's studies. *Social Sci. Med.* 1985; **21**: 985–96.

23. Forbes, J.F., McGregor, A. Unemployment and mortality in postwar Scotland. *J. Health Econ.* 1984; **3**: 239–57.

24. McAvinchy, I.D. Unemployment and mortality: some aspects of the Scottish case 1950–78. *Scot. J. Polit. Econ.* 1984; **31**: 827–53.

25. Warr, P. Twelve questions about unemployment and health. In: Roberts, R., Finnegan, R., Gallie, D., eds. *New approaches to economic life.* Manchester: Manchester University Press, 1985.

26. Moser, K.A., Fox, A.J., Jones, D.R., Goldblatt, P.O. Unemployment and mortality: further evidence from the OPCS longitudinal study 1971–81. *Lancet* 1986; **i**: 365–6.

27. Moser, K.A., Goldblatt, P.O., Fox, A.J., Jones, D.R. Unemployment and mortality: comparison of the 1971 and 1981 longitudinal study census samples. *Br. Med. J.* 1987; **294**, 86–90.

28. Ruberman, W., Weinblatt, E., Goldberg, J.D., Chaudhary, B.S. Psychosocial influences on mortality after myocardial infarction. *N. Engl. J. Med.* 1984; **311**: 552–9.

29. Spruit, I.P. *Unemployment, employment, and health.* Leiden: Leiden University, 1983.

30. Svensson, P.G. *International social and health policies to prevent ill health in the unemployed—the World Health Organisation perspective.* Copenhagen: WHO, 1983.

31. Mitchell, J.R.A. Hearts and minds. *Br. Med. J.* 1984; **289**: 1557-8.

32. Black, D., Morris, J.N., Smith, C., Townsend, P. *Inequalities in health. The Black report.* Suffolk: Chaucer Press, 1982.

33. Wilkinson, R.G. *Class and health: research and longitudinal data.* London: Tavistock, 1986.

34. Walker, A., Noble, I., Westergaard, J. *From secure employment to labour market insecurity: the impact of redundancy on older workers in the steel industry.* Sheffield: University of Sheffield, 1983.

7

'I couldn't stand it any more'
Suicide and unemployment

A 40-year-old Welshman hanged himself after searching unsuccessfully for work for 10 months. The next day a letter arrived offering him a job. The letter the dead man left said: 'I can't go on like this, reading and watching television all day. I'm drinking my unemployment money away.' Was it unemployment or poverty that led this man to kill himself, or was it alcohol? Or was it a combination of all three, or none of them?

Such questions are impossible to answer, but even the most casual readers of British newspapers will have noted accounts of inquests where coroners have suggested that people (almost always men) have killed themselves because they could not find jobs. The journalist John Pilger selected 12 such stories from 'a much longer list' collected between June 1983 and June 1984.[1] These accounts do not impress scientists much because there is no proof that unemployment caused these men to kill themselves, but they do impress the public; and they may thus have a bigger effect on politicians than scientific studies because, when the chips are down (and an election is in the offing), politicians pay much more attention to public opinion than to scientists.

But scientists have devoted considerable energy to studying the relation between suicide and unemployment, and Platt has collected no fewer than 156 relevant studies in a review that is unlikely to be superseded for some time.[2] Unemployment has been associated not only with suicide but also with the inelegantly named parasuicide, which the *Oxford Textbook of Medicine* prefers to call 'non-fatal deliberate self harm' and define as 'a deliberate non-fatal act, whether physical, drug overdosage, or poisoning, done in the knowledge that it was potentially harmful, and in the case of drug overdosage, that the amount taken was excessive'.[3] Despite the preference of the Oxford textbook, I will use the word 'parasuicide'—as do most people writing on the subject. But it is important not to be deceived by the similarity of the words 'suicide' and 'parasuicide' into thinking that parasuicide is simply failed suicide: it is not. Suicide is usually associated with severe and often long-standing psychiatric or physical illness and is commoner in older people and in men; parasuicide, in contrast, is commoner in younger people and women and is usually not associated with long-standing psychiatric illness, although the patients have often experienced intense but short-lived anxiety or depression. Parasuicide, too, is commoner in social classes IV and V and in deprived urban areas: some association with unemployment would thus be expected.

Studies looking for an association between suicide and unemployment are much commoner than those looking for an association with parasuicide, and the main reason for this is simply that parasuicide is a modern phenomonen: it has increased rapidly in the past 20 years and now accounts for about a fifth of all medical emergency admissions. (Interestingly, the most recent data suggest that the parasuicide rate has begun to fall, while the unemployment rate has continued to rise.) Although the older studies have thus been of suicide and unemployment, many recent studies are of parasuicide. These have the potential to be more rewarding: because there are many more cases of parasuicide than suicide prospective studies of individuals become a possibility and also the individuals are left alive to investigate. Nevertheless, these potential advantages have not led to much. And one disadvantage is that parasuicide is more difficult both to define and to measure than suicide.

More than 150 years ago Falret suggested that suicide rates rise during economic depressions,[4] and Durkheim (who gave us the very modern word 'anomie') in his classic book on suicide confidently wrote: 'It is a well known fact that economic crises have an aggravating effect on the suicidal tendency.'[5] But many contemporary researchers are less confident.

In his review Platt follows Dooley and Catalano[6] in classifying studies of unemployment and both suicide and parasuicide into cross-sectional versus longitudinal, and individual versus aggregate. For each condition there are four possible categories of study: individual cross-sectional, aggregate cross-sectional, individual longitudinal, and aggregate longitudinal. This is not an entirely happy classification and the jargon is intimidating, but the system is worth following because it provides some guide to a maze of often inadequate and contradictory studies.

Many uncontrolled studies of suicides have found high unemployment rates, and two recent case-control studies have found significantly more unemployment among men who have killed themselves than among matched psychiatric controls.[7, 8] Roy looked at 90 psychiatric patients (53 men and 37 women) who had killed themselves and found that 38 of the men (72 per cent) were unemployed compared with 23 (43 per cent) of the psychiatric controls ($p < 0.02$).[7] The difference was not significant among the women, and Robin et al., although they found significantly more unemployment among men who had killed themselves, found that among women more of the controls (5/50) than the cases (1/50) were unemployed.[8] This may be something to do with the difficult problem of classifying unemployment among women (is a woman with two children under three years old unemployed because nobody pays her?).

Platt found four studies that looked at suicide rates among the employed compared with the unemployed: generally rates are higher among the unemployed. But again the association is not so strong for women.[9-12] Studies like these cannot tell us whether unemployment is leading to suicide or whether a psychiatric illness that leads to unemployment also leads to suicide. Some of these cross-sectional

---

It's made me very quick tempered. I lose my temper just like that [he snaps his fingers]. I get bored very easily. I prefer to be on the go all the time. If I got a job I'd want to do it every hour of the day if I could, to stop me being bored. Just loafing about gets right up my nose. You can't even watch TV in the day, there's nothing on for the unemployed. As time goes on, I've got very pessimistic about getting another job. You reach the point where you get to the door of the interview and you say to yourself, what a waste of bloody time. The Jobcentre is useless: you spend quite a lot of time looking till you find a job you really like, you think great, then you get the girl to phone up. But it's always gone. It's really heartbreaking. You pick out any card you like in there, and I'll guarantee you won't get that job because it will be gone.

PAUL HARRISON An unemployed deaf man quoted in *Inside the Inner City* [Harmondsworth: Penguin, 1983]

studies of suicide and unemployment have looked at the 'cause' of unemployment and several mention poor physical or mental health.[13, 14] Others have attempted retrospectively to work out how much unemployment contributed to death, and only one was unequivocal that it had; however, the paper did not give adequate data to support the conclusion.[15]

Cross-sectional studies of whole populations, which compare suicide rates and unemployment rates in different geographical areas (wards, boroughs, counties, or countries), are even less helpful. Some show a positive correlation, others show a negative one, and most find no significant relation.

Platt found eight studies that looked at individuals and used a longitudinal design.[16-23] Three were retrospective and found some association between suicide and unemployment or occupational loss.[16-18] One British study looked at the work records of 40 men and 35 women who had killed themselves and compared them with those of 150 controls matched by age, sex, location, and marital status.[18] At the time of death significantly more of the cases than the controls were unemployed (9 versus 0) or off sick (6 versus 4), and in the three years before death 95 per cent of the controls had either kept the same job or changed it only once, compared with 66 per cent of the cases. Of the nine patients who had killed themselves when unemployed, two had been dismissed (one for drinking) and seven had left voluntarily (five impulsively and two because they could not keep up with the work).

The other five individual longitudinal studies are prospective, but none is the perfect study that would have detailed and validated information on the health of a large employed group representative of the general population and then closely followed it for years so that the work records of those who eventually killed themselves could be compared with the records of those who did not. Because suicide is a rare event, such a study could probably never be mounted. The study that comes closest is that of the Office of Population Censuses and Surveys that I described in the last chapter: it showed a statistically significant association between unemployment and suicide, but the authors could not be confident either that poor mental health had not led to both unemployment and suicide or that some other confounding variable such as educational status, housing, or alcohol problems had not accounted for the association.[19] The

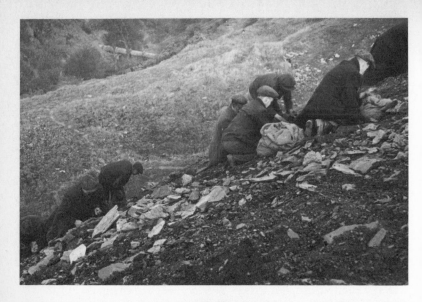

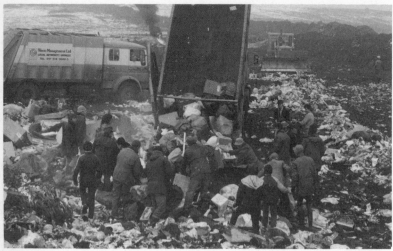

PLATE 7.1 Top: unemployed men scratch for coal at a slag heap in Newcastle, December 1938 (copyright BBC Hulton Picture Library). The picture was used by the Germans in the last war to illustrate the terrible conditions that existed in Britain. Below: unemployed men search for saleable objects among the waste being dumped at Bidston Moss, Merseyside, 1985 (photograph by Peter Marlow, copyright Magnum). Jack describes the scene: 'These are people up to their shins every day in old tea bags, cat food tins, and onion skins, sliding and falling on slopes of polythene bags and bacon rind, scrambling to get a copper wire before the next man, seizing a pair of discarded shoes, triumphantly unearthing a bicycle pump, shouting a warning when the municipal bulldozer threatens to bury half a dozen of them in a grave of discarded nylon stockings and fish finger cartons.' [Life on the scrap heap]. *Sunday Times Colour Magazine* 1985; 19 May: 26-31]

preliminary analysis of the data from the 1981 census show a standardized mortality ratio for suicide among those seeking work of 241 (95 per cent confidence interval 93–458).[24] The standardized mortality ratio for the whole 10 years of the earlier study was 273 (95 per cent confidence interval 159–416). So the pattern is looking the same.

Two large Scandinavian prospective studies of psychiatric patients related the work experience of those who eventually killed themselves to matched controls, but they found contradictory results.[20, 21]

The largest number of unemployment and suicide studies have been aggregate longitudinal studies which look for an association between unemployment rates (or other indicators of economic recession) and suicide rates over time. Most of the 30 studies find a positive correlation; indeed, all but one of the 22 American studies do.[2] Durkheim's confidence was thus not too misplaced, but evidence from Britain is more conflicting. Swinscow found a positive correlation between unemployment and suicide in Britain for 1923–47,[25] but Kreitman and Platt found a significant negative correlation among men for 1955–80.[26] Cleverly, however, they discovered that this negative association arose in the eight-year spell 1964–72 and hypothesized that it had something to do with the introduction of natural gas in Britain. Kreitman had argued previously that this had been the cause of the significant fall in suicide from carbon monoxide poisoning,[27] and once suicides from domestic gas poisoning had been excluded from the analysis there was a significantly positive correlation between suicide and unemployment in Britain for 1955–80.[26]

Many studies have reported on unemployment rates among patients seen after parasuicide. Whenever comparisons are possible the rates seem to be higher than those among the general population. The first cohort studies of patients who had deliberately harmed themselves—from Edinburgh and Newcastle in the early 1960s—showed that about a third of the men were unemployed, and this proportion has had a tendency to rise ever since.[28, 29] In 1982 in Edinburgh 62 per cent of the 501 men seen after parasuicide were unemployed, as were 47 per cent of the 213 seen in Oxford (unpublished data quoted by Platt[2]).

Studies that have compared parasuicide rates among the unemployed and the employed have tended to show much higher rates among the unemployed.[30, 31] Kessell *et al*. showed that in a provincial region of Victoria, Australia, the parasuicide rate per 100 000 men for 1971-2 was 21 for professionals and managers, 109 for white collar workers, 234 for blue collar workers, and 2686 for the unemployed.[31] In Edinburgh, Platt and Kreitman found that the rate per 100 000 men for 1968 was 98 for the employed and 2824 for the unemployed, a ratio of nearly 29 to 1 (see Table 7.1).[32] The ratio of relative risk was linked strongly to length of unemployment: it was 9 to 1 among those unemployed for fewer than 4 weeks; 5 to 1 among those unemployed for 5 weeks to 6 months; 10 to 1 among those unemployed for 6 to 12 months; and 19 to 1 among those unemployed for more than a year. These figures fit with one of the 'phases' models of unemployment, which suggests that the initial shock of unemployment causes much distress and that people then adapt only to become steadily more distressed if they do not find a job after many months.

Thus the evidence is strong that many of those who are seen after parasuicide are unemployed and that the risk of parasuicide is much higher among the unemployed than the employed. Oddly, however, unemployment is rarely mentioned by the unemployed as a cause of their injuring themselves.[33-35] Almost always the main precipitating event is a row or a fight with a loved one. But these results do not mean that unemployment is unimportant in leading to parasuicide, for it is axiomatic that there is a considerable gap between why we think and say we do things and the 'real' reason why we do them. Also unemployment may make people more likely to injure themselves but may only rarely be what precipitates the injury—most, after all, have been unemployed for more than six months when they injure themselves.

Aggregate cross-sectional studies of unemployment and parasuicide have been carried out in Edinburgh[36, 37] and in Brighton.[38] These studies have shown a positive and significant association between unemployment and parasuicide—that is, areas with more unemployment tend to have more parasuicide. There are also strong associations with other indicators of poverty and deprivation.

No good individual longitudinal study of parasuicide and unemployment has been carried out, although such a study might be possible with parasuicide because it is so much commoner than suicide. (Platt disagrees and suggests that a prospective cohort study

TABLE 7.1. Incidences of parasuicide among employed and unemployed men in Edinburgh city and measures of relative and population attributable risk, 1968–82

Year	Incidence of parasuicide/100 000			Relative risk ratio*	Population attributable risk†	Maximum percentage of overall incidence attributable to unemployment‡
	Among unemployed	Among employed	Among all economically active			
1968	2824	98	172	29.0	74	43.2
1969	2284	117	188	19.6	71	38.1
1970	1955	122	204	16.1	82	40.4
1971	2302	115	238	20.0	123	51.5
1972	2106	141	252	14.9	111	44.0
1973	2458	134	240	18.3	106	44.2
1974	2374	149	247	15.9	98	39.6
1975	1991	139	239	14.4	100	42.1
1976	2052	173	299	11.8	126	42.0
1977	1779	153	284	11.6	131	45.9
1978	1647	150	257	11.0	107	41.8
1979	1523	160	253	9.5	93	36.6
1980	1663	143	260	11.6	117	45.0
1981	1743	154	322	11.3	168	52.3
1982	1345	114	272	11.8	158	57.8

* Parasuicide incidence among the unemployed to parasuicide incidence among the employed.
† Parasuicide incidence among all economically active men minus parasuicide incidence among employed men.
‡ Population attributable risk divided by parasuicide incidence among all economically active men.

is not practicable or feasible.[2]) There have, however, been aggregate longitudinal studies of parasuicide and unemployment from Edinburgh[32] and Oxford.[39]

The Edinburgh study showed overall a strong positive association between parasuicide and unemployment rates among men for 1979–82 (Table 7.1)[32, 37]—although this association broke down in 1982 and has puzzlingly been negative for 1983 and 1984 (S. Platt, personal communication). The fall in the relative risk of parasuicide among the unemployed compared with the employed may, the authors hypothesize, be due to more mentally healthy people finding themselves unemployed when overall unemployment is high. When unemployment is low the selection effect, whereby the unhealthy are more likely to lose their jobs, may be more powerful. Platt and Kreitman also found that the relative risk of parasuicide was lower in those areas of Edinburgh with high unemployment: this may be because the stigma of unemployment is less in such areas. This fits with a further finding that the relative risk is highest in social classes I and II, despite both unemployment and parasuicide being much commoner in lower socioeconomic groups. In a rather sad way these last results might be seen as optimistic: once unemployment becomes very common in particular groups, then the misery is reduced.

The data from Oxford also show a correlation between unemployment among men and the proportion of employable men who were unemployed when they injured themselves: the risk of parasuicide was about 12 to 15 times higher among the unemployed than among the employed.[39] The risk of parasuicide was also related to duration of unemployment, being 26 to 36 times higher among those unemployed for more than a year than among the employed. Hawton and Rose from Oxford looked too at the psychiatric and alcohol histories of the unemployed who injured themselves and found that, compared with the employed, twice as many had been in psychiatric care (a quarter as against one in ten were receiving psychiatric treatment at the time, and alcoholism was diagnosed three times more often).

Clearly both suicide and parasuicide are associated with unemployment. The unemployed are over-represented among both people killing and non-fatally injuring themselves, and suicide and parasuicide rates are higher among the unemployed than among the employed. Most longitudinal studies of individuals show more unemployment and job instability among those who kill or injure

---

Two men who go every day to the dump at Bidston Moss (see Plate 7.1) describe the experience:

'I couldn't believe it when I came here first. For the first two weeks I just stood here and looked at them. Well, I'd never been out of work before and never seen anything like it. But there's not much else you can do, you know what I mean? Just now the kids' bedroom needs redecorating. I could never afford the paper and paint on social security. This way you earn a bit extra, but I still can't stand the shite and the dogs. You get about half a dozen dead dogs up here every day. And cats. People just put them into plastic bags. Even now if I come across shite or a dead dog, that's it. I just walk down the road and go home for the day.

'You come every day and meet your mates. It's like a proper job. It's so boring being unemployed. I eat, breathe, and sleep tip. I'd still come if I won the pools. It's part of life, getting your hands dirty, isn't it?'

[Ian Jack in 'Life on the scrap heap.' *Sunday Times Colour Magazine* 1985; 19 May: 26-31]

---

themselves non-fatally, and all aggregate studies from the United States show that unemployment and suicide rates have changed together. The seemingly inconsistent results from Britain in the 1960s can, with considerable confidence, be attributed to the introduction of natural gas.

But the question remains: How is unemployment associated with suicide and parasuicide? Although there is good evidence that unemployment causes deterioration in mental health, it does not prove that unemployment on its own causes either suicide or parasuicide. The other possible explanations are that people with poorer mental health are more likely to become unemployed, or that both the higher unemployment and suicide and parasuicide rates are caused by other factors—for instance, poverty or alcohol problems.

The answer is almost certainly that all three explanations contribute. Those in poorer health seem to be more likely to become unemployed and find it more difficult to get another job. The mental health of most people suffers during periods of unemployment and continues to deteriorate as the time without work continues. And these miseries are associated with poverty, unhealthy changes in lifestyle, poor education, bad housing, and other factors that may contribute to higher suicide and parasuicide rates.

There will be no simple explanations. Students of medicine and particularly of epidemiology seem to find themselves grappling with problems that are ever more complex and ever more resistant to their traditional methods of study. The epidemiology of smoking-related disorders is more complicated than the epidemiology of cholera. And the epidemiology of disorders associated with alcohol is more complicated than both: the range of conditions associated with alcohol is wider; the data on which hypotheses must be generated and tested are weaker; there are more confounding variables; the latest round of concern with the issue is newer; and the problem is just more complicated. The epidemiology of unemployment and health is more complicated still, for essentially the same reasons.

References

1. Pilger, J. Death on the dole. *Daily Mirror* 1984; July 10: 12–14.

2. Platt, S. Unemployment and suicidal behaviour: a review of the literature. *Social Sci. Med.* 1984; **19**, 93–115.

3. Morgan, H.G. The patient who has attempted suicide. In: Weatherall, D.J., Ledingham, J.G.G., Warrell, D.A., eds. *Oxford textbook of medicine.* Oxford: Oxford University Press, 1983.

4. Falret, J.P. *De l'hypochondrie et du suicide.* Paris, 1822.

5. Durkheim, E. *Suicide.* London: Routledge and Kegan Paul, 1897.

6. Dooley, D., Catalano, R. Economic change as a cause of behavioural disorder. *Psychol. Bull.* 1980; **87**: 450–68.

7. Roy, A. Risk factors for suicide in psychiatric patients. *Arch. Gen. Psychiat.* 1982; **39**: 1089–95.

8. Robin, A.A., Brooke, E.M., Freeman-Browne, D. Some aspects of suicide in psychiatric patients in Southend. *Br. J. Psychiat.* 1968; **114**: 739–47.

9. Sainsbury, P. *Suicide in London.* London: Chapman and Hall, 1955.

10. Yap, P.M. Suicide in Hong Kong. *J. Mental Sci.* 1958; **104**: 266–301.

11. Cumming, E., Lazar, C., Chisholm, L. Suicide as an index of role strain among employed and not employed married women in British Colombia. *Can. Rev. Social Anthropol.* 1975; **12**: 463–9.

12. Kraft, D.P., Babigian, H.M. Suicides by persons with and without psychiatric contacts. *Arch. Gen. Psychiat.* 1976; **33**: 209–15.

13. Stearns, A.W. Suicide in Massachusetts. *Mental Hygiene* 1921; **5**: 752–77.

14. Tuckman, J., Lavell, M. Study of suicide in Philadelphia. *Public Health Rep.* 1958; **73**: 547-53.

15. Sathvayathi, K. Suicide among unemployed persons in Bangalore. *Ind. J. Social Work* 1977; **37**: 385-92.

16. Humphrey, J. Social loss: a comparison of suicide victims, homicide offenders, and non-violent individuals. *Dis. Nervous System* 1977; **38**: 157-60.

17. Olsen, J., Lajer, M. Violent death and unemployment in two trade unions in Denmark. *Social Psychiat.* 1979; **14**: 139-45.

18. Shepherd, D.M., Barraclough, B.M. Work and suicide: an empirical investigation. *Br. J. Psychiat.* 1980; **136**: 469-78.

19. Moser, K.A., Fox, A.J., Jones, D.R. Unemployment and mortality in the OPCS longitudinal study. *Lancet* 1984; **ii**: 1324-9.

20. Hagnell, O., Rorsmann, B. Suicide in the Lundby Study: a controlled prospective investigation of stressful life events. *Neuropsychobiology* 1980; **6**: 319-32.

21. Borg, S.E., Stahl, M. Prediction of suicide: a prospective study of suicides and controls among psychiatric patients. *Acta Psychiat. Scand.* 1982; **65**: 221-32.

22. Cobb, S., Kasl, S.V. Some medical aspects of unemployment. *Industrial Geront.* 1972; **8**: 8-15.

23. Theorell, T., Lind, E., Floderus, B. The relationship of disturbing life changes and emotions to the early development of myocardial infarction and other serious illnesses. *Int. J. Epidemiol.* 1975; **4**: 281-93.

24. Moser, K.A., Goldblatt, P.O., Fox, A.J., Jones, D.R. Unemployment and mortality: comparison of the 1971 and 1981 longitudinal study census samples. *Br. Med. J.* 1987; **294**: 86-90.

25. Swinscow, D. Some suicide statistics. *Br. Med. J.* 1951; **i**: 1417-22.

26. Kreitman, N., Platt, S. Suicide, unemployment and domestic gas detoxification in Great Britain. *J. Epidemiol. Community Health* 1984; **38**: 1-6.

27. Kreitman, N. The coal gas story: UK suicide rates 1960-71. *Br. J. Prev. Social Med.* 1976; **30**: 86-93.

28. Kessel, N. Self poisoning—part I. *Br. Med. J.* 1965; **ii**: 1265-70.

29. Kessel, N. Self poisoning—part II. *Br. Med. J.* 1965; **ii**: 1336-40.

30. Whitlock, F.A., Schapira, K. Attempted suicide in Newcastle-upon-Tyne. *Br. J. Psychiat.* 1967; **113**: 423-34.

31. Kessell, A., Nicholson, A., Graves, G., Krupinski, J. Suicidal attempts in an outer region of metropolitan Melbourne and in a provincial region of Victoria. *Aust. N.Z. J. Psychiat.* 1975; **9**: 255-61.

32. Platt, S., Kreitman, N. Trends in parasuicide and unemployment among men in Edinburgh, 1968–82. *Br. Med. J.* 1984; **289**: 1029–32.

33. Morgan, H.G., Burns-Cox, C.J., Pocock, H., Pottle, S. Deliberate self-harm; clinical and socioeconomic characteristics of 368 patients. *Br. J. Psychiat.* 1975; **127**: 364–74.

34. Smith, J.S., Davidson, K. Changes in the pattern of admissions for attempted suicides in Newcastle-upon-Tyne during the 1960s. *Br. Med. J.* 1971; **iv**: 412–15.

35. Shapiro, C.M., Parry, M.R. Is unemployment a cause of parasuicide? *Br. Med. J.* 1984; **289**: 1622.

36. Buglass, D., Duffy, J.C. The ecological pattern of suicide and para-suicide in Edinburgh. *Social Sci. Med.* 1978; **12**: 241–53.

37. Platt, S., Kreitman, N. Parasuicide and unemployment among men in Edinburgh, 1968–82. *Psychol. Med.* 1985; **15**: 113–23.

38. Bagley, C., Jacobson, S., Palmer, C. Social structure and the ecological distribution of mental illness, suicide, and delinquency. *Psychol. Med.* 1973; **3**: 177–87.

39. Hawton, K., Rose, N. Unemployment and attempted suicide among men in Oxford. *Health Trends* 1986; **18**: 29–32.

8

'I'm just not right'
The physical health of the
unemployed

MEDICINE'S bias is towards physical rather than psychological illness: in his training a doctor spends most time studying physical illness, and he will often go to great lengths to exclude a physical cause for a patient's symptoms even though he is convinced that the cause is psychological. Readers may therefore be surprised that this chapter on the physical health of the unemployed comes after the one on their psychological health. But this reversal of the usual bias reflects the superiority of research into unemployment and psychological health compared with that into physical health.

Despite Britain having more than three million unemployed people nobody has ever started the large longitudinal study that would have been needed to tell us exactly how unemployment affects physical health or, indeed, how much more at risk those in poor physical health are of becoming unemployed. The best large studies that we have—those from the Office of Population Censuses and Surveys longitudinal study[1] and from the British Regional Heart Study[2]—are both spin-offs from studies undertaken for other reasons; both therefore offer only partial insights into the problem. And the best of the smaller studies—that from a general practice in Calne, Wiltshire[3]—was undertaken because of the general practitioner's enthusiasm, not because anybody in government was concerned to know the effect of unemployment on physical health.

The failure to start a high-quality study of this problem is an indictment of politicians, doctors' leaders, and those who decide research priorities. Whether nobody saw the need for such a study or whether a study was proposed and rejected because of the political sensitivity of unemployment I do not know, but a variety of people around the country have suggested to me that the government has discouraged rather than encouraged research into unemployment and health.

One prospective longitudinal study that did produce information was done in Michigan in the 1970s. It is often quoted because it was for a long time the only well-designed and, more importantly, controlled study.[4-8] The study was, however, small and the initial field work was done in 1967, when unemployment was not nearly as severe as now; and most of the 113 men made redundant got other jobs quite quickly. Cook and Shaper have said that the results are less interesting than the methods, and they suggest that it should be thought of as a pilot study.[9] Unfortunately nobody has satisfactorily repeated the study despite almost 20 years passing and unemployment becoming a much bigger problem all round the world.

I have already described the design and some of the results of the Michigan study in Chapter 5 (p. 72). The researchers used many different measures of health, including a 'days complaint score', a symptoms scale, and a depression score (many of these measures did not produce satisfactory results). The researchers also measured blood pressure and serum concentrations of cholesterol and uric acid.

The researchers found no significant changes in blood pressure among the controls from just under two months before the plants closed until two years after. Nevertheless, among the men made redundant there was a significant drop in systolic (5.32 mmHg) and diastolic (3.06 mmHg) blood pressure from the early phase, when they were expecting redundancy, were unemployed, or just starting new employment, to the later phase, when most were settled in new jobs. Unfortunately the researchers have no data from before closure was mooted, but they show a significant increase in both systolic and diastolic blood pressure as closure came closer. They also showed that those whose blood pressures remained high longer had more difficulty finding a permanent job. Although these data may be statistically significant, they are of doubtful clinical importance, and there were too few men who could be classed as hypertensive to allow statistical analysis. Another flaw is that the nurses who took the blood pressure knew which men had been made redundant, although, as the authors point out, they did not have records of their previous measurements and it is the change that is being measured. For all these reasons the results cannot be seen as very important.

The sick versus the unemployed role

Sick	Unemployed
Exempted from certain social obligations and commitments	Not exempted from social commitments; expected to fulfil them irrespective of financial and emotional problems
Cannot voluntarily recover or be held responsible for his condition	Expected to be able to recover and held responsible if he cannot find work
Must want to get well and be willing to seek and accept treatment	Must regard unemployment as undesirable and temporary and must accept work of any type and at any wage
Continuation depends on becoming a patient and accepting competent (professional) help	If he does not find a job he is deemed lazy or incompetent and 'has something wrong with him'
Can be granted only if there is adequate evidence of internal disease	Permanent unemployed status granted only if there is evidence of unemployability—chronic disease, total abandonment, or demoralization

Another report from the Michigan study showed that uric acid but not cholesterol concentrations were higher in men expecting closure of the plants than in controls.[5] The uric acid concentrations dropped sharply to normal when men found new jobs quickly, but otherwise remained high until men settled into new jobs. Cholesterol concentrations rose when men became unemployed and dropped later when they found jobs. Again the methods are more interesting than the results because the clinical importance of these results is not clear. They show that statistically significant bodily changes can be detected in people experiencing redundancy and unemployment and that these changes are reversed with re-employment, but whether such changes are important remains unknown. The poverty of the conclusions is well illustrated by a sentence from a later report on the study: 'In a larger sample an excess of diabetes, peptic ulcer, and

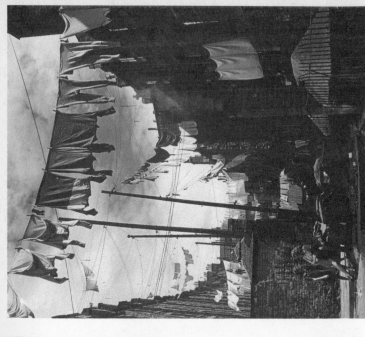

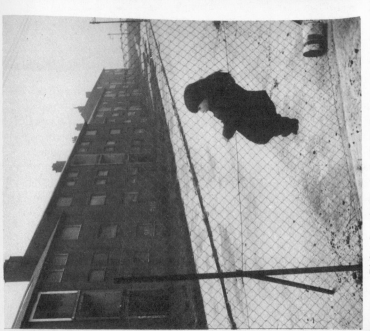

PLATE 8.1 Right: slums in Dundee in the 1940s (photograph and copyright W. Suschitzsky) and (left) in Glasgow in 1985 (copyright International Freelance Library).

gout might appear and there may have been a temporary increase in atherogenesis which might have future implications.' (This reminds me of a notice I once saw in a tobacconist's window advertising 'a small miniflatlet'.)

Clinically more important results have come from the British Regional Heart Study.[2] Detailed information was collected from January 1978 to June 1980 on 7735 men aged 40–59 who were randomly selected from representative general practices in 24 medium-sized British towns. No inner city areas were included and only two of the towns, Hartlepool and Merthyr Tydfil, had high unemployment. The men were asked various questions about employment, including 'If you are unemployed is this because of ill health?' On the strength of their answers the men were classified into employed (7165), ill unemployed (258), not ill unemployed (150), retired (55), and unemployed but not clearly ill or not ill (7). Thus 5.3 per cent of the men were unemployed, which is lower than the national average at the time and much lower than the present 13 per cent. As would be expected, the unemployed were slightly older and less skilled than the employed.

Although the authors do not make much of it, I find it surprising and interesting that 63 per cent of the unemployed and 76 per cent of the 259 who had been unemployed for more than a year should say that they were unemployed because of ill health; and some of those who had retired had also probably done so because of poor health. Probably some men answered yes to the question because the stigma of being sick is much less than the stigma of being unemployed—the 'sick role' is much preferable to the 'unemployed role' (box, p. 115).[10] Indeed, in response to my articles published in the *British Medical Journal* a woman wrote to describe how demeaning it is for an unemployed person who has a working spouse and no dependants because he or she is not then entitled to any other benefit after becoming ineligible for unemployment benefit: 'My husband', she wrote, 'was one of the lucky ones whose unemployment made him very ill.'[11] He then became eligible for sickness benefit.

When such a high percentage of those without jobs say that they have lost them because of ill health it is no wonder that there are powerful associations between unemployment and ill health. But as unemployment increases, so broader categories of workers—for example, the skilled as well as the unskilled and the healthy as well as

the ill—lose their jobs, and so the association between unemployment and ill health may weaken.

The men in the Regional Heart Study were asked whether their
doctors had diagnosed any of 12 illnesses (angina, heart attack, other
heart trouble, high blood pressure, stroke, diabetes, peptic ulcer,
gout, gall bladder disease, thyroid disease, arthritis, bronchitis, and
asthma). They were also asked standard questions to determine
whether they might have bronchitis or ischaemic heart disease.
Their blood pressure was measured, and they completed simple lung
function tests.

About half the employed (49 per cent), the unemployed who were
not ill (47 per cent), and 82 per cent of the ill unemployed recalled
that their doctors had diagnosed at least one illness. The screening
showed that both the groups of unemployed were more likely to
suffer from bronchitis, obstructive lung disease, and ischaemic heart
disease, even after standardization for age, social class, town of
residence, and smoking state. The higher prevalence compared with
the employed was significant for all conditions in the ill employed
but only for ischaemic heart disease in the not ill unemployed. For
hypertension there were no significant differences.

This study does not allow conclusions on whether unemployment
causes ill health or vice versa, but the authors hoped that the information that would continue to emerge from the study would lead to
more confident conclusions. Indeed, they sent the men in the study a
questionnaire asking about work experience and promised an analysis
linking the answers to the health information that they had gathered.
But five years have past since the original report and no further
information has appeared. Why? Is it because somebody somewhere
doesn't want any more information to emerge? I have no evidence to
support this conspiracy theory, but that such an opportunity should
be wasted is a great shame.

Yet another study that was not specifically designed to answer
questions on health and unemployment but which did produce some
information was the Department of Health and Social Security
cohort study.[12] It was started in response to public worries about
'scroungers' and the worry that some people were better off on the
dole than in work (very few were). A national sample of 2300 men
who became unemployed in the autumn of 1978 was asked questions
relevant to health one, four, and twelve months after registration:

12 per cent of the sample was unemployed for the whole year. Among the whole sample 12 per cent had spent some time out of work sick in the year before the study began, and among those who were unemployed for the whole year 22 per cent had spent time sick. Older men were both more likely to have been out of work sick and to have been continuously unemployed. During the year of the study only 8 per cent of the sample had time off sick, which might be interpreted as representing an improvement in health. But the fall may well be due, the authors warn, to under-reporting of sickness because of the 'time and effort' necessary to move from unemployment benefit to sickness benefit and back again.

The men were also asked whether they had a disability or a health problem, and at the first interview 19 per cent said that they had. Again the proportion increased with age: 9 per cent among those under 25 to 38 per cent among those aged 50–59. During the year of the study 18 per cent of those who said that they had a disability remained continuously unemployed compared with 11 per cent of those without a disability. Nevertheless, at each interview the proportion reporting a disability or health problem remained about the same. Again, there is no evidence of an increase in self-reported health problems. At the second and third interviews the men were asked whether their health had stayed the same, got better, or got worse. About three quarters at both interviews said that it had stayed the same, and roughly equal numbers said that it had got better or worse.

The authors 'cautiously' conclude that if there is an effect of unemployment on health then it is small: there was little decline in health even among those unemployed for the whole year. Also most people who become unemployed are healthy and stay that way, but those who start with a disability are more likely to stay without a job and so the long-term unemployed will contain a higher proportion of the unhealthy. Another conclusion is that the 'sick' among the employed are not a static group.

The caution is because there was no control group, and the information was all self-reported; the study lasted for only a year and was small, and there was attrition in the sample from the original 2300 to 1500 by the third interview. These limitations are so severe that the study might be disregarded but for the fact that we do not have much that is better; the authors conclude that 'the effect of unemployment

My husband is disabled but seeks work. He has been out of work a number of years. I also have a son just left school who is out of work. He is not the type of lad who does not seek work. He has a pile of letters—about 70 to be precise—about jobs he has written off for. We have got to the point where if we see a van with an address on he jots it down and he writes off. There are no vacancies but he might be lucky one of these times. We have to live with not enough money for the things other people take for granted, such as a weekend joint. This is a luxury for us. Our weekend joint is strips of breast of lamb, turkey wings, or even a tin of corned beef. We survive on stodge such as potatoes, rice. Chips are a main meal with egg. The unemployed take a lot of stick. They are made out to be scroungers and weak people. It's not them, it's the system. We treat as luxuries what other people take for granted—good meals, nice clothes, holidays—and just being able to buy something without thinking what will I have to do without to buy this item. And it's always thinking, 'No, I don't really need it.' And you always walk away feeling really low. You feel let down, full of stress, ratty with the family and friends. I dread Christmas coming on.

JENNIE POPAY Extract from a letter quoted in *Unemployment and the Family* [London: Unemployment Alliance, 1984]

on health will be . . . a fruitful area for future research'. There is little evidence that the department that sponsored the research has heeded this conclusion.

Further, and again limited, information comes from the United Kingdom Training Survey—a complicated statistical analysis of the remembered work experience of 17 707 men who were available for work from 1965 to 1975.[13] The authors concentrated on those who were either 'sick' or 'unemployed' for over three months, trying to work out whether such an experience increased the probability of another such experience. A spell of sickness, they concluded, made another such spell more likely, as did an experience of three months or more of unemployment, but there was little evidence that a spell of unemployment made sickness more likely.

The limitations of this study were that no information was given on sample selection, all the information was based on recall, and three months was a long time to be unemployed in 1965–75.

People do not visit their doctors only when they are sick, and many people who are sick do not seek professional help. However, we can

ethodological weaknesses. In Chapter 6 I concluded
uld not be certain, although we could be fairly confident,
ployment caused extra and premature deaths. Similarly,
t be certain that unemployment causes extra physical
hough the best evidence suggests that it does. As a group
ployed are, however, more unhealthy than the employed
y the unhealthy have a higher chance of becoming and
nemployed.

es

K.A., Fox, A.J., Jones, D.R. Unemployment and mortality in
gitudinal study. *Lancet* 1984; **ii**: 1324-9.

D.G., Cummins, R.O., Bartley, M.J., Shaper, A.G. Health of
ed middle-aged men in Great Britain. *Lancet* 1982; **i**: 1290-4.

N., Nethercott, S. Job loss and family morbidity: a study of factory
R. Coll. Gen. Pract. 1985; **280**: 510-14.

S., Cobb, S. Blood pressure changes in men undergoing job loss: a
ry report. *Psychosom. Med.* 1970; **32**: 19-38.

S.V., Gore, S., Cobb, S. The experience of losing a job: reported
n health, symptoms and illness behaviour. *Psychosom. Med.* 1975;
21.

S.V., Cobb, S., Brooks, G.W. Changes in serum uric acid and
ol levels in men undergoing job loss. *J. Am. Med. Ass.* 1968; **206**:

, S., Kasl, S.V. *The consequences of job loss.* Washington: US Depart-
Health, Education and Welfare, 1977.

, S. Strategies of research on economic stability and health. *Psychol.*
82; **12**: 637-49.

, D.G., Shaper, A.G. Unemployment and health. In: Harrington,
. *Recent advances in occupational health.* Vol II. Edinburgh: Churchill
tone, 1985.

in, L., Little, M. *The forsaken families.* Harmondsworth: Penguin,

w, M. Occupationless health. *Br. Med. J.* 1985; **291**: 1506.

ylan, S., Millar, J., Davies, R. *For richer, for poorer? DHSS study of
oyed men.* London: HMSO, 1984.

get more information on how unemployment affects health by
looking at how those without jobs—and their families—use health
services. Warr has summarized several aggregate studies from
America that have searched for associations between hospital admission rates and unemployment, and they produce conflicting
evidence.[14] Some authors who have found increases in hospital
admissions in association with unemployment think that the mechanism is more that unemployment 'uncovers' illness rather than
'provokes' it; thus the health services may be more accessible to
the unemployed, they may have more time to attend, or they may
feel less able to cope with usual illnesses.[15, 16] Some authors have
suggested that unemployment may be associated with reduced visits
to doctors and hospitals because those who are just clinging on to
jobs may be reluctant to go sick.[14, 17]

The DHSS cohort study showed that the unemployed used health
services more than the general population, as measured from the
General Household Survey, but the authors did not control for
disability or for socioeconomic status.[12] The study also showed that
the long-term unemployed did not consult general practitioners
more often than the short-term unemployed.

Jacobsen, in contrast, studied the workers at a factory that had
closed and found that those who lost their jobs sought medical advice
significantly more often in the month in which the factory closed and
in the following month than they did in the same months in the
previous year.[18]

Three controlled studies have all shown that the unemployed
consult their doctors more often than the employed.[3, 19, 20] One of
these was a prospective study of 300 men aged between 35 and 60
and living in Miami. Linn *et al.* identified 30 who had lost their jobs
but had not been fired. They then followed them up and compared
their health with 30 closely matched controls. At the beginning of
the study—in 1979—the two groups had similar psychological and
physical health, but over the next six months the unemployed were
significantly more likely to suffer a deterioration in mental health
(although there was a wide range in response, with some improving)
and significantly more likely to see their doctor, spend days sick in
bed, and take medicines. In six months the employed visited their
doctors 1.2 times on average, whereas the unemployed visited 5.9
times. The unemployed, however, had on average almost exactly the

same number of diagnoses made (1.9) as the employed (1.8). The study also showed strong correlations between measures of psychological and physical health: the lower the degree of social support of the unemployed man and the lower his self-esteem, the more likely he was to visit his doctor.

This is an important study but a small one. Furthermore, the authors do not know how stressful were the jobs the unemployed lost, and as the study began after the men had lost their jobs nothing is known about when the changes in health began. Nor, because of the short follow up, do the authors know if the unemployed men will adapt the longer they are unemployed.

A large controlled—but cross-sectional—study from Canada also showed that the unemployed used health services more often than the employed.[20] The Canada Health Survey gathers data on 12 000 households using interviews, self-administered questionnaires, and examinations by doctors. In the unemployment study, results are given for 14 313 people over 15 (including women), 1803 (12.6 per cent) of whom were unemployed. The unemployed visited their doctors on average 3.4 times a year compared with 2.55 times for the employed ($p < 0.001$). This was particularly true of those from higher socioeconomic groups and those with more education. They also had significantly more short-term and long-term disability, and significantly poorer mental health on a number of measures. Examination by the doctors showed that the unemployed had significantly more heart trouble, pain in the heart and chest, spells of fainting and dizziness, high blood pressure, and bone and joint problems ($p < 0.001$ in all cases). Interestingly, the study showed no significant difference in tobacco or illicit drug consumption, but the employed drank more alcohol than the unemployed.

Although it might seem unlikely, one of the best studies on unemployment comes from rural Wiltshire—from Calne. For a great many years the small town was dominated by a large sausage factory, but now the factory has gone, to be replaced by a big hole. Sometime after the factory closed a general practitioner, Norman Beale, whose practice was right beside the factory, began to wonder what effect the closure might have had on the practice. He rather thought that consultation rates might have gone down. The factory workers who had been injured had often come quickly to the practice and demanded to be seen. Beale began to study what had happened, and the study that

began in this small way has now [...] importance.[3] Beale has described the [...] truth.[21]

Together with Susan Nethercott, [...] from his practice 80 men and 49 w[...] when the factory closed. They then l[...] of the workers and their families fron[...] closed, and they plan to continue u[...] factory finally closed in 1982). Very [...] their jobs have moved away. Compar[...] and 22 women) the families of those [...] significant 20 per cent increase in thei[...] time they knew the factory might close—[...] until two years afterwards.[3] Visits to hos[...] also increased by 60 per cent—despite t[...] miles away—and these may be more like[...] consultations to be for definable phy[...] Nethercott point out that if similar inc[...] families of the 3.3 million unemployed p[...] must be considerable costs to the Nationa[...]

Beale and Nethercott then went on t[...] particularly at risk and found that olde[...] before the threat of redundancy had con[...] quently were the ones who increased their[...] Men and women who exhibited both of th[...] a 150 per cent increase in the number of co[...] increase in number of episodes of illness, a[...] in the number of attendances at outpatient[...]

These important increases would, how[...] unnoticed in the average practice. 'A thi[...] number of consultations by the . . . older [...] observe Beale and Nethercott, 'results in a [...] only 0.32 per cent in a practice of 11 300. M[...] their jobs these employees consulted 57 per [...] during the previous year. Such is the futility[...] polls of family doctors for credible evidence [...] dancies in their communities cause ill health[...]

The studies discussed here have produced [...] on how unemployment might affect physical [...]

severe n[...] that we c[...] that une[...] we cann[...] illness, a[...] the unen[...] and clea[...] staying u[...]

Referen[...]

1. Mose[...] OPCS lo[...]

2. Cook[...] unemplo[...]

3. Beale[...] closure.[...]

4. Kasl,[...] prelimin[...]

5. Kasl[...] changes [...] **37**: 106[...]

6. Kasl [...] choleste[...] 1500-7[...]

7. Cob[...] ment o[...]

8. Kas[...] *Med.* 1[...]

9. Coc[...] J.M., e[...] Living[...]

10. Fa[...] 1984.[...]

11. Sh[...]

12. M[...] *unemp*[...]

13. Narendranathan, W., Nickell, S., Metcalf, D. An investigation into the incidence and dynamic structure of sickness and unemployment in Britain, 1965-75. *J. R. Statis. Soc.* 1985; **148**: 254-67.

14. Warr, P. Twelve questions about unemployment and health. In: Roberts, R., Finnegan, R., Gallie, D., eds. *New approaches to economic life.* Manchester: Manchester University Press, 1985.

15. Dooley, C.D., Catalano, R., Jackson, R., Brownell, A. Economic life and symptom changes in a non-metropolitan community. *J. Health Social Behav.* 1981; **22**: 144-54.

16. Ahr, P.R., Gorodezky, M.J., Cho, D.W. Measuring the relationship of public psychiatric admissions to rising unemployment. *Hospital Community Psychiat.* 1981; **32**: 398-401.

17. Higgs, R. Unemployment in my practice. Walworth. *Br. Med. J.* 1981; **283**: 532.

18. Jacobsen, K. Dismissal and morbidity. *Ugeskrift Laeger* 1972; **134**: 352-4.

19. Linn, M.W., Sandifer, R., Stein, S. Effects of unemployment on mental and physical health. *Am. J. Pub. Health* 1985; **75**: 502-6.

20. D'Arcy, C., Siddique, C.M. Unemployment and health: an analysis of 'Canada Health Survey' data. *Int. J. Health Serv.* 1985; **15**: 609-35.

21. Beale, N. From brainwave to breakfast television. *Br. Med. J.* 1986; **292**: 869-70.

22. Job loss and health—the influence of age and previous morbidity. *J. R. Coll. Gen. Pract.* 1986; **36**: 261-4.

9

'We got on each other's nerves'
Unemployment and the family

LESS than 5 per cent of Britons live in the story-book family with two dependent children, a father who is working, and a wife who stays at home,[1, 2] but most of us continue to live with other people, and the unemployment of one family member can affect all the others and the functioning of the whole. Hypotheses and anecdotes abound on how unemployment may damage, or rarely enhance, family life, but good research and hard evidence are less common. The whole subject of unemployment and health is under-researched, but the particular topic of the effect of unemployment on family life and health may be the most poorly researched of all—despite unemployment and family life both being at the centre of the political stage. Or perhaps it is because they are so politicized that we know so little about them.

In 1984 about 1.3 million British children were growing up in families where the main breadwinner was unemployed.[3] Of those 206 000 were living in homes where the breadwinner had been unemployed for one to two years, and 536 000 in homes where he or she had been unemployed for more than two years.[3] Over half (53 per cent) of all unemployed men are aged between 18 and 34, the ages when most start their families, and among the 801 000 men who have been unemployed for over a year the proportion rises to 61 per cent—486 000 men.[4] In 1982, according to the General Household Survey, just under half (49 per cent) of unemployed men were married, and just under a third (29 per cent) had dependent children: 9 per cent had one child, 11 per cent had two, and 5 per cent had three.[5] In 1980, among those unemployed for over a year and aged between 25 and 44 almost two thirds (64 per cent) had dependent children, and in December 1982, 622 000 long-term unemployed claimants were responsible for almost half a million children.[6] It must be remembered, too, that many families contain dependants who are not children. One small survey in the north east showed that there were more carers (almost always women) looking after elderly, frail, and handicapped relatives than mothers looking after children under 16.[6]

How many wives and mothers are unemployed is hard to say because of the difficulty of interpreting the unemployment figures for women: many do not register as unemployed because they are not entitled to benefits or are seeking only part-time work. Many more who might like a job might not even consider looking for one—either because they don't think they would get one or because 'there are people more deserving of one'. Women are under increasing pressure to stay at home. Nevertheless, many cannot stay at home, either because the woman working is the only way to keep a two-parent family out of poverty, or because the woman has no partner: more than one in eight families is headed by only one person, and in almost 90 per cent of cases this is a woman.[2]

This difficulty in classifying the employment status of women is one of the main reasons for the inadequacy of the research into the effects of unemployment on women.[7] (Many feminists would argue that sexism in research is just as important.) An example of the difficulties of classification is provided by the important Office of Population Censuses and Surveys longitudinal study of unemployment and mortality. Women were excluded because those who described themselves as 'seeking work' were a small and select group, and 38 per cent of the women in the sample aged 15–59 were 'placed in the inactive category to which housewives were allocated'.[8] Another study published in the same year illustrates further the confusion over women and employment as well as showing how health researchers are still more preoccupied with the harmful effects of work rather than of its absence.[9] Although they do not say so specifically, Murphy *et al.* were clearly primarily interested in whether paid employment might be bad for pregnant women. They looked at 20 613 married women who had their first babies in Cardiff, Barry, or Penarth between 1965 and 1979—79 per cent were employed during pregnancy, and the other 21 per cent were classed as non-employed. The non-employed are not classified further, however, and presumably include two very different groups: women who wanted work but could not get a job and women who may have

My wife, she don't respect me any more. My son, Abdul, asked me so many times for a push bike, and I said, 'Son, as soon as I get a job I will buy a bike, and please don't play with the neighbour's push bike.' I can't maintain, can't buy presents for my son. I couldn't bring presents for my son Haru's birthday. I can't buy shoes, as I am expected. My wife's sister came from Pakistan, and I am unable to take them to Blackpool, to show the seaside. They spent a lot of money to come down here, they pay the milk bills. This makes me feel bad. I am happier that they return, because I don't feel shame, because they spend their money. Indira treats me differently. If I ask her to do a job before, she does it. Nowadays, she says she will do it later on. She criticises me, she thinks I'm responsible. If I don't get a job she says, 'Why didn't you get it?' So I say, 'It's not my fault.' When I first lost my job she said I was unlucky. She was praying that I get a job. Children were also sad, because I couldn't pay for things. When I was working, Indira and the children and me used to go out shopping together. Now I go on my own for the groceries.

LEONARD FAGIN and MARTIN LITTLE An unemployed Asian man, who had been a leading hand and shop steward in a factory making washing machines, quoted in *The Forsaken Families* [Harmondsworth: Penguin, 1984]

chosen not to work—perhaps for the benefit of their unborn baby. It is thus hard to make sense of the findings that the perinatal outcome was significantly better among the employed women and that the non-employed women were more likely than the employed to be at the extremes of maternal age, to have a history of medical problems and previous abortions, and to attend less often for antenatal care. Unemployment among the non-employed women may well have caused or contributed to their poorer outcomes, and in that context it is interesting that women in social classes I and II were at greater risk than those in lower social classes.

One factor that emerged from this Welsh study was that non-employed women were more likely than employed women to be married to unemployed men. This fits with other evidence from the General Household Survey that unemployment is concentrated in the same families, which goes not only for husbands and wives but also for children.[6] A government survey from 1977 showed that one in seven unemployed people had fathers out of work and 20 per cent had an unemployed brother or sister,[6] and a small-scale survey in 1982 of participants in the community industry scheme found that almost a third of unemployed young people had one or both parents unemployed.[10]

One of the main ways in which unemployment harms families is through poverty. In its first report in 1982 the Social Security Advisory Committee said that unemployed claimants with dependent children 'must include people who are among the worst off of all supplementary benefit claimants. Families are found to encounter all sorts of pressing needs for additional spending after spending a year on benefit'.[11] Poverty is most acute among the long-term unemployed because unemployment benefit stops after a year and the unemployed are not eligible for the long-term supplementary benefit rate. The Advisory Committee in its second report said: 'It is manifestly wrong to us that they [the unemployed] should be expected to live on some £10.60 a week (1983 prices) less than pensioner couples . . . when they are already at a level of income where differences of pence, let alone pounds, can matter deeply.'[12]

The average couple with two children spent about £149 a week on everything except housing in 1983, and at the same time rates of benefits for a family of the same size were £59.20.[13] Unemployed families complain more about financial difficulties than anything else, and there is much evidence of parents going without so that their children can be adequately clothed and fed.[6, 14, 15] The mother of one unemployed family told a researcher: 'We've made do with a piece of toast, we've always had our main meal at night, always. We've never gone without that have we, even if it's only egg and chips. But perhaps we've had a piece of toast dinner time instead of having a normal meal so the children can have theirs. We usually find that at the end of the fortnight.'[15]

Economic factors are important in determining marriage and birth rates, and during recessions both marriages and births tend to decline. During the 1930s in Britain and Australia crude marriage rates fell and the average age of both men and women at first marriage rose.[16, 17] The same picture has emerged in the recent recession.[5, 18] Birth rates tend naturally to vary with marriage rates, and they have fallen during the recent recession, as they did in the 1930s. Windschuttle has looked at the Australian data and declared himself satisfied that unemployment and recession are having an important effect on the Australian family, but I know of no statistical studies correlating unemployment with marriage and birth rates. We cannot be confident that unemployment in itself, and particularly prolonged unemployment, leads to reductions in births and marriages.

The contradictions in how unemployment may affect marriage and reproduction emerge in small descriptive studies. Popay quotes a 19-year-old Liverpudlian who had been unemployed since leaving school as saying that because he had no job he couldn't contemplate having a girlfriend, getting married, and raising a family—and he didn't think that he would ever get a job.[6] He would never have a 'normal family life'. Campbell, in contrast, notes that 'unemployed girls who've never experienced economic independence are doing the only thing they can—having babies, either getting married or not. . . . They never consider an abortion, often don't use contraception. They want children. Of course they do.'[19] Beale and Nethercott noticed a significant rise in the pregnancy rate compared with controls among women laid off when the sausage factory in Beale's practice in Calne, Wiltshire, closed: four of six women who were married, aged under 30, and without children and who were laid off conceived in the next 21 months compared with ten of 54 controls ($p = 0.02$).[20] The authors conclude their short paper with the question; 'If large numbers of unemployed women are allowing themselves to fall pregnant by a process of "negative" family planning—"I may as well . . ."—will it precipitate an increase in rejection of infants, puerperal mental illness, and child abuse?'

Burgoyne surveyed 100 married couples in which the man was unemployed and found that 70 per cent of them said that unemployment made no difference to their decisions on starting or adding to their families, while 23 per cent said it had put them off and 7 per cent said it had encouraged them.[21] In her intensive study of 17 young families McKee found that for most of them the husband's employment status was of little or no consequence in the decision when to start a family.[15] Many pregnancies happened accidentally, and more important than the man's employment was the age of the mother, the existing family size, the mother's employment status, the age and sex of existing children, and the duration of the marriage. These factors are, of course, those that are important in employed families, and McKee concludes that families want to do what seems 'normal' to them. One woman said: 'People say to me you shouldn't have children in this industrial climate, but I don't think that way.

And I'd like another even now, even if I'm out of work, 'cause if all the unemployed stopped reproducing . . . you'd have workers having children and unemployed not.'[15]

Deciding whether or not to become pregnant and then whether to go forward with the pregnancy is complex, and many factors are important. Nevertheless, a man's unemployment may play a crucial if not decisive part in the decision—as one woman's story illustrates. She became pregnant soon after her husband had lost his job: 'It really depressed me . . . it all seemed to come together, being pregnant, people getting at Paul [her husband], and it took it out of me. I went to the doctor, I was on tranquillisers. I got so depressed. I suppose it was having three other children and then having Kay, 'cos she wasn't planned. I went to have an abortion. The thing was with Paul being on the dole there was no way we could afford another baby. And I went to the hospital and couldn't go through with it.'[15]

Whether or not it leads to more children who may not be 'wanted' unemployment can destroy relationships just as it destroys individuals. The deterioration in the mental health of the unemployed person—be it the father, the mother, or a child—affects his or her relationships with the rest of the family. And in this time of misery the family are likely to be thrown together more, usually in financially reduced circumstances, and sooner or later something may snap.

Divorce rates have surged in Britain since 1971, when the Divorce Law Reform Act came into force, and so it is hard to sort out longitudinally the influence of unemployment on marital breakdown. But cross-sectional data show that the divorce rate in 1979 among unemployed men aged 16–59 was 34 per 1000 while among all men of that age it was 15.[22] For all age groups the divorce rate of the unemployed was double that of the national average. These figures do not, of course, prove that unemployment is causing marital breakdown, but they are very suggestive. Burgoyne found that a third of her 100 couples had reported a deterioration in their relationship, compared with only 3 per cent of matched control couples.[21] About half of the couples reported an increase in arguments, and in a third one or other partner had either contemplated leaving or had left temporarily. Another small but intensive study was carried out by Judith McLellan, a health visitor, in an inner city area in the north west of England where unemployment was 42 per cent.[23] She looked at 20 unemployed families, and in 16 both partners agreed that their relationship had deteriorated since the unemployment began. Five of the couples had also experienced physical aggression for the first time since unemployment began. In one case a husband insisted that his wife have an abortion for a 10-week pregnancy because they could not afford another child.

Wife battering and child abuse (particularly sexual abuse) have come much more into the public eye during the same time that unemployment has increased, and many people and politicians have assumed that they are therefore cause and effect. Similar assumptions have been made about unemployment causing drug taking, street violence, and crime, but it is wrong to move from correlations to assumptions about causation—after all, the number of colour television sets in Britain has also increased considerably in the last 10 years. Yet it seems likely that there might be a link between unemployment and domestic violence and child abuse.

A study of 100 cases of wife battering published in 1975, when male unemployment in Britain was about 5 per cent, found that 48 per cent of the husbands or cohabitees had been unemployed at some time and 29 per cent were frequently or mostly unemployed.[24] Other factors that were associated with the battering included heavy drinking, gambling, and a prison record. Similar results have emerged in Australia, where 45 per cent of the husbands of women presenting to the Elsie Women's Refuge, Sydney, in 1975 were unemployed—a rate 26 times higher than the Australian average at the time.[17] The Australian Royal Commission on Human Relationships in 1976 invited battered wives to 'phone in', and among the 56 women who gave their husband's employment status 13 (23 per cent) had husbands who were unemployed.[17] Windschuttle attributes the differences in the results to the socioeconomic variation in the two groups: most of the callers to the Royal Commission were from higher socioeconomic groups, among whom unemployment was lower. One woman who rang the commission said: 'When he lost his job he went absolutely bonkers. He changed completely. He became depressed and snappy. Frustrated.'[17]

The British study[24] reported an association between wife battering and child abuse, and the parallelism of the curves showing an increase in unemployment and prevalence of child abuse has struck researchers. The figures of the National Society for the Prevention of

Cruelty to Children show that the rate of children being physically injured began to rise dramatically in 1979 and increased by half over the next three years.[25] Since then—particularly since the media have taken a great interest in the subject—the increase has been even more dramatic. (I am not arguing that the media have created the problem but rather that many cases that went unreported are now being brought to light.) Cases of child abuse presenting to paediatricians in Leeds trebled between 1979 and 1984 after remaining stable for the four years before.[26] At the same time the number of cases of sexual abuse increased from none to 50. The author of this study produces no evidence that unemployment was the cause, but he is struck by the fact that it was 1979 when unemployment began to increase dramatically in Britain. The factors most often mentioned as precipitating the abuse to 6532 children registered with the National Society for the Prevention of Cruelty to Children between 1 January 1977 and 31 December 1982 were unemployment, marital discord, debts, and parents' lack of self-esteem.[25] Unemployment itself leads to debts, lack of self-esteem, and marital discord.

Fathers of children notified to the society in 1976 had an unemployment rate six times that of the general population,[27, 28] and a study in Dundee found that almost a third of the fathers of abused children were out of work.[29] A nationwide American study found that the fathers and mothers of abused children had poor employment records, and at the time of the incident 12 per cent of the fathers were unemployed—three times the national rate at the time.[30] Steinberg et al. have moved on from these cross-sectional studies to do an aggregate longitudinal study over 30 months in two distinct metropolitan communities. They showed that increases in child abuse were preceded by periods of high job loss, and they were confident that the two were cause and effect.[31] At the other end of the methodological spectrum McLellan in her study found that 11 of her 20 couples reported a deteriorating relationship with their children, and six admitted to having physically assaulted their children.[23] Children taken into care—not all of whom are abused—are also likely to have unemployed parents: in one small study in 1976 almost half of the parents of children taken into care were unemployed.[32]

The health of the children of the unemployed may be harmed in ways other than by violence or neglect, and some evidence points to

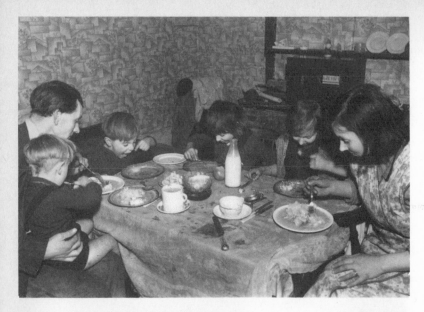

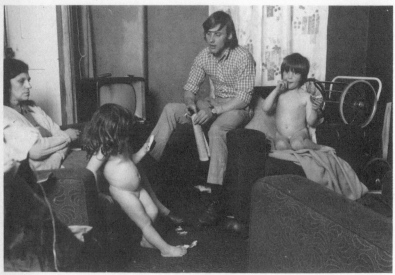

PLATE 9.1 Unemployed families in the 1930s (top) and 1970s (below). (Both pictures copyright BBC Hulton Picture Library.)

higher mortality rates. Infant and neonatal mortality declined in the 1930s (although maternal mortality increased) and perinatal mortality has declined since 1976, which inclines politicians towards the view that unemployment in particular and recession in general cannot have much effect on infant deaths.[33] The 1985 figures for Scotland, however, show a small increase in perinatal mortality,[34] and specific studies have suggested an association between unemployment and perinatal and infant mortality.[33]

An analysis of data from the 1971 census showed a positive association between death rates of children aged 0 to 4 years and unemployment rate, low socioeconomic status, and inadequate and overcrowded housing, and the unemployment rate seemed to have an effect independent of class.[35] Deaths in children aged 5–14 years were not associated with unemployment. Another study of all deaths in Sheffield in children aged 8 days to 2 years between April 1979 and April 1981 found a significantly greater number of adverse social factors (including unemployment) in 15 children dying of potentially preventable conditions compared with children dying of conditions with a poor prognosis, those who presented as unexplained cot deaths, and controls.[36] Interestingly, the effect seemed to be independent of social class. Only one study has used data from the 1981 census, finding a strong association in 30 postal districts of Glasgow between unemployment and admission rates of children to hospital.[37]

The survey of all births in one week in April 1971 has been used to look for associations between unemployment and outcome of pregnancy as questions were asked in the initial survey about the employment status of both the mother and the father; questions were also asked about intervening employment in the follow-up in 1975.[38] A study of 15 000 singleton pregnancies showed that within each class women married to unemployed men compared with women whose husbands had jobs made less use of contraceptives, had had more babies, attended fewer antenatal clinics and classes, smoked more, and were less likely to breast feed. All of these are risk factors associated with a poor outcome for the pregnancy, but, although there was a 50 per cent excess risk of perinatal death among the babies born to unemployed fathers, the increase did not reach statistical significance.[33] This may well have been because of the small size of the study and the low rate of unemployment, and the study cries out to be repeated today when unemployment is so much higher.

Large studies need to be done when studying perinatal death, because death is comparatively rare. Studies of birthweight are easier, and birthweight is known to be an important risk factor for perinatal death. A study of 655 Glasgow babies showed that after adjusting for other factors the mean birthweight of those with unemployed fathers was 150 g less than that of those with employed fathers.[39] A longitudinal study of 107 babies from either a richer or a poorer area showed that the 2.6 per cent deficit in growth in the first year in those from the poorer area was completely explained by adjusting for length at 1 month, father's height, and whether the father was employed.[39] A study of 20 600 Dublin babies showed that those born to unemployed fathers had a mean birthweight 20 g lower than those born into social class V and 80 g lower than those born into social class IV.[40] The Glasgow researchers suggested that their study had produced some evidence that unemployment among men was causally related to growth faltering in their babies, and said that it was important that a national study of trends in birthweight during the years of rapid increase in unemployment be done. Such a study hasn't yet been done and probably never can be, because the years of rapid rise are over.

Stein *et al.* identified in a prospective study of 483 pregnant women 14 babies with low birthweight (under 2500 g) and 14 who were delivered preterm (before 37 weeks).[41] Five of the 14 women giving birth to a baby of low birthweight had an unemployed partner—a significantly higher proportion than those who gave birth to a baby of normal weight (60/457) ($p < 0.05$). The women with an unemployed partner were not more likely, however, to deliver prematurely. In contrast to other studies, social class, adverse life events, and psychiatric status were not associated with giving birth to a baby of low birthweight, although a low income was—which may reflect the small size of the study.

Two national studies of child growth since 1972 have shown that the children of the unemployed tend to be shorter than those whose fathers are employed, and this effect is greatest in the children of the long-term unemployed.[42, 43] The preschool growth study has also found that at 2 years of age the children of the unemployed are significantly more likely to fail developmental tests; this was not so at age 1.[44, 45, 46] tsmouth Social Services Research and Intelligence Unit. *Children on* . Portsmouth: Portsmouth Social Services Research and Intelligence 976.

cfarlane, A., Cole, T. From depression to recession—evidence about cts of unemployment on mothers' and babies' health, 1930s-1980s. ward, L., ed. *Born unequal: perspectives on pregnancy and childrearing ployed families*. London: Maternity Alliance, 1985.

onymous. Infant mortality rises in Scotland. *Br. Med. J.* 1985; **291**:

nnan, M.G., Lancashire, R. Association of childhood mortality with status and unemployment. *J. Epidemiol. Community Health* 1978; 33.

/lor, E.M., Emery, J.L. Family and community factors associated ant deaths that might be preventable. *Br. Med. J.* 1983; **287**: 871-4.

clure, A., Stewart, G.T. Admission of children to hospitals in /: relation to unemployment and other deprivation variables. *Lancet* : 682-5.

lding, J., Thomas, P., Peters, T. Does father's unemployment put us at risk? Quoted in: Macfarlane, A., Cole, T. From depression to n—evidence about the effects of unemployment on mothers' and health, 1930s-1980s. In: Durward, L., ed. *Born unequal: perspectives nancy and childrearing in unemployed families*. London: Maternity , 1985.

e, T.J., Donnet, M.L., Stanfield, J.P. Unemployment, birth weight, wth in the first year. *Arch. Dis. Child.* 1983; **58**: 717-21.

wding, V.M. New assessments of the effects of birth order and socio- ic status on birth weight. *Br. Med. J.* 1981; i: 683-6.

n, A.L., Campbell, E.A., Day, A., Cooper, P.J. Social adversity, low ight, and preterm delivery. *Br. Med. J.* 1987 (in press).

a, R.J., Swan, A.V. Altman, D.G. Social factors and height of school children in England and Scotland. *J. Epidemiol. Community* 978; **32**: 147-54.

ional Study of Health and Growth. *Report*. London: Social e and National Health Services Research Unit and Division of nity Health, St Thomas's Hospital Medical School, 1984.

artment of Health and Social Security, Subcommittee on Nutritional ance. *Report of Health and Social Subjects*. London: HMSO, 1981.

nnock, A., Keegan, P.T., Fox, P.T., Elston, M.D. Associations be- rowth patterns, social factors, morbidity, and developmental delay in

We know remarkably little about how the unemployment of a male breadwinner affects the general health of a family, and we know even less about the effect of unemployment on a wife when the husband is still in work. Moser *et al.* have shown from the OPCS longitudinal study an increase in the mortality of wives of unemployed men[8] and in that of other women (daughters, for instance) living in the same household.[47] Beale and Nethercott have shown a significant increase in both the consultation rates and referral rates to hospital of whole families when redundancy threatens.[48] Fagin and Little in their small uncontrolled study found that some wives became depressed, especially if they were not working and were dependent on their husband's working image, and they also found in the children of three of their families an increase after the father's job loss of dis- turbances in feeding habits, minor gastrointestinal complaints, sleep- ing difficulties, proneness to accidents, and behaviour disorders.[49] McLellan found new illness in many of the wives in her study of 20 families, and four women, she thought, needed hospital treatment.[23] Fourteen of the couples reported 51 new problems in 29 children. Twelve aged between 3 and 11 developed behaviour problems; seven aged between 4 and 10 began to wet the bed; and seven aged 6 to 14 began to fail at school.

A study just as small—but controlled—from North Carolina found that in the 18 children of workers made redundant, there was a sig- nificantly higher incidence of episodes of illness and days sick with all illnesses including infection than among the 13 children of retained workers. Haggerty in an anniversary discourse to the New York Academy of Medicine described a study in which among 100 people in 16 families the frequency of infection with streptococci was sig- nificantly related to the degree of chronic stress, of which unemploy- ment was one of the main causes.[50]

Despite what the reader may think, this is not an impressive haul of evidence. Many small and rather poorly designed studies have been done, but more should have been done. If I stop to think of the amount published on, for instance, hypertension or cancer of the colon, I can conclude only that doctors and medical researchers have shamefully neglected the study of how unemployment harms the health of families. For it seems wholly likely that family life is shaken by unemployment—often to the point of disintegration—and we have evidence that points towards possible increases in divorce, domestic violence, abortions and unwanted pregnancies, perinatal and infant mortality, and morbidity in wives and children, as well as evidence of failure of growth in children. Although none of the evidence provides us with the degree of proof that reluctant politicians (sometimes) demand before they will take action, almost all of it points in the direction of unemployment seriously harming families as well as individuals.

References

1. Longfield, J. *Ask the family: shattering the myths about family life.* London: Bedford Square Press/National Council for Voluntary Organizations, 1984.

2. Family Policy Studies Centre. *The family today: continuity and change.* London: Family Policy Studies Centre, 1984.

3. Family Policy Studies Centre. *Family trends and social security reform.* London: Family Policy Studies Centre, 1986.

4. Anonymous. Labour market data. *Employment Gazette* 1986; December: S1-S68.

5. Anonymous. *General household survey 1982.* London: HMSO, 1984.

6. Popay, J. *Unemployment and the family.* London: Unemployment Alliance, 1984.

7. Popay, J. Woman, the family, and unemployment. In: Close, P., Collins, R., eds. *The family and economy in modern society.* London: Macmillan, 1985.

8. Moser, K.A., Fox, A.J., Jones, D.R. Unemployment and mortality in the OPCS longitudinal study. *Lancet* 1984; ii: 1324-9.

9. Murphy, J.F., Dauncey, M., Newcombe, R., Garcia, J., Elbourne, D. Employment in pregnancy: prevalence, maternal characteristics, perinatal outcome. *Lancet* 1984; i: 1163-6.

10. Shanks, K., Courtenay, G. *Young people, work and community industry.* London: Community Industry, 1982.

11. Social Security Advisory Committee. *Annual report 1982.* London: HMSO, 1983.

12. Social Security Advisory Committee. *Annual report 1983.* London: HMSO, 1984.

13. Roll, J. Better benefits for babies—financial support for pregnancy and unemployment. In: Durward, L., ed. *Born unequal: perspectives on pregnancy and childrearing in unemployed families.* London: Maternity Alliance, 1985.

14. Salfield, A., Durward, L. 'Coping but only jus[t] of pregnancy and childrearing on the dole. In: [*unequal: perspectives on pregnancy and childrearing* London: Maternity Alliance, 1985.

15. McKee, L. 'We just sort of struggle on'—havin[g] unemployment. In: Durward, L., ed. *Born unequal: and childrearing in unemployed families.* London: M[

16. Office of Population Censuses and Surveys[London: OPCS, 1977:23.

17. Windschuttle, K. *Unemployment: a social an[d economic crisis in Australia.* Ringwood, Victoria: P[

18. Office of Population Censuses and Surveys. [HMSO, 1984.

19. Campbell, B. *Wigan pier revisited.* London: V[

20. Beale, N., Nethercott, S. Job loss and first pre[*Br. Med. J.* 1986; 292: 799.

21. Burgoyne, J. Unemployment and married life. [1985; November: 7-10.

22. Central Statistical Office. *Social Trends* 1985;[

23. McLellan, J. The effect of unemployment on [1986; 58: 157-61.

24. Gayford, J.J. Wife battering: a preliminary su[*J.* 1975; ii: 388-91.

25. Creighton, S.J. *Trends in child abuse.* London[Prevention of Cruelty to Children, 1984.

26. Wild, N.J. Sexual abuse of children in Lee[ds 113-6.

27. Madge, N. Annotation: unemployment and [*Child Psychol. Psychiat.* 1983; 24: 311-9.

28. Creighton, S.J. *Child victims of physical abu[Society for the Prevention of Cruelty to Childre[

29. Cater, J., Easton, P. Separation and other s[1980; i: 972-3.

30. Gil, D.G. *Violence against children: physica[States.* Cambridge, Mass.: Harvard University P[

31. Steinberg, L.D., Catalano, R., Dooley, D[child abuse and neglect. *Child Dev.* 1981; 52: 9[

a longitudinal survey of preschool children. In: Borns, J., ed. *Human growth and development*. London: Plenum, 1984.

46. Fox, P.T., Hoinville, E.A. Current social factors and the growth of preschool children. *Proc. Nutr. Soc.* 1984; **43**: 79A.

47. Moser, K.A., Fox, A.J., Jones, D.R. Goldblatt, P.O. Unemployment and mortality: further evidence from the OPCS longitudinal study 1971-81. *Lancet* 1986; **i**: 365-6.

48. Beale, N., Nethercott, S. Job loss and family morbidity: a study of a factory closure. *J. R. Coll. Gen. Pract.* 1985; **35**: 510-4.

49. Fagin, L., Little, M. *The forsaken families*. Harmondsworth: Penguin, 1984.

50. Haggerty, R.J. Stress and illness in children. *Bull. N. Y. Acad. Med.* 1986; **62**: 707-18.

10

'What can be done?' Responding to unemployment and health

THE first 10 of the articles that have been revised to form this book, the ones which assembled the evidence on unemployment harming health, were published some months before the four articles that discussed how the problem might be tackled. The commonest response that I had from doctors and other health workers to the first series of articles was 'They are so sad, but what can we do?' I too—before I began my research—tended to be rather pessimistic and thought that reducing the number of unemployed was the only answer—and what could health workers or individuals do about that?

Now I recognize that much can be done, and at all levels. Governments have a part to play, but so do health authorities, local authorities, industry, trade unions, employers, and individuals. What I also recognize—through reading the work of those who have written on the future of work and employment[1-6]—is that we are at a threshold. Either we will enter a nightmare in which the unemployed will grow in numbers and poverty while those with employment resort increasingly to armies and policemen to keep them safe, or we will enter a world in which the dream of being relieved of alienating toil is realized, employment is shared out, and we think very differently about work. Many of us would not be so rich in material terms, but we would have recognized that unpaid work can be just as (and often more) rewarding than paid employment. This might sound rather fanciful, and the two options I describe are the extremes, but the possibility that by the year 2000 three out of four jobs could be done by machines[2] opens up these options. Probably we will end up with something of both options, but these broad-brush futures should, I believe, be kept in mind as we consider more immediate responses to the misery of unemployment.

These final chapters will draw together the many initiatives that have either been tried or proposed. I will start from 'the top' and work down, hoping that those who feel that 'nothing can be done' will be led to think again.

Reducing unemployment is the obvious way of attacking the problem, and even this is not just for politicians and businessmen because organizations and individuals—including doctors—can take on new employees, either on their own initiative or through the various Manpower Services Commission programmes. In addition, the work that is available can be shared out more fairly, and this policy too can be pursued by individuals as well as governments. Then, although decently paid employment is what people want most now, voluntary work is better than nothing. Health authorities and doctors know how much 'work' needs to be done to help lonely, sick, and disabled people—and they should be able to bring together those who need work and those who need help.

Other strategies try to reduce the harm done by unemployment, and one of the most potent ways of doing this is to reduce the poverty of those who have no job. Politicians (and doctors and other health workers) can argue for increased and better distributed benefits, but individuals can also work to increase the number who claim the benefits to which they are already entitled; few people are better placed to do this than doctors. They can also point their unemployed patients towards the vast array of statutory and voluntary schemes that offer retraining, counselling, education, advice on leisure, ideas on job creation, practical help, companionship, and stimulation. Health and social workers can also offer themselves and their time, and, although they have no pills with which to treat unemployment, they can show that they understand and care. Such 'treatment' might do much to ameliorate the apathy, pain, and humiliation of prolonged unemployment.

Health workers can also lead the way in reducing the stigma attached to unemployment. Too many of those in 'comfortable' Britain have no understanding of what it is like to be unemployed and how difficult it is for those who have been without jobs for long periods to sustain their self-esteem and find decent jobs. There is far too much talk of scroungers. Health workers must recognize that unemployment may strike almost anybody and damage their health, and they can help to bring home that fact to those lucky enough to have jobs.

Mr Geoffrey Holland, the director of the Manpower Services Commission, said recently: 'It has been the devil's own job to get people concerned about long-term unemployment. There is warm individual and collective support for helping young people, but it is only in the last year or so that the public has become aware of the problems of long-term unemployment.'[7]

What is needed is a blueprint for action at every level, and already plans have been made. The European office of the World Health Organization has a strategy for counteracting the health damage caused by unemployment,[8] although its book on targets for health in Europe by the year 2000 hardly mentions unemployment, despite the first aim being to reduce inequalities in health by 25 per cent.[9] The health departments of various governments—including, for instance, the Swedish—have also adopted plans.[10] (Unemployment in Sweden is around 3 per cent.)

The Association of Metropolitan Authorities has looked at the implications for the authorities in caring for the unemployed,[11] and

---

CHARTER FOR **JOBS**

We believe that the present level of unemployment is economically wasteful and socially corrosive. The government can and must stimulate the creation of more jobs.

There is useful work crying out to be done. With extra spending we could renovate our cities and improve the health of our people, while lower taxes on jobs would raise private spending power and make us more competitive. To make this possible there has to be some increase in government borrowing. Government borrowing should normally rise in a depression. When there is useful work to be done, it is as sensible for the government to borrow money as for firms or families to do so.

The government has a special responsibility for the million and a quarter people who have been unemployed for over a year. These people should be guaranteed the offer of a job on socially useful projects, such as the Community Programme supports.

Formed last year to lobby the government to create new jobs, Charter for Jobs has representatives from all the main political parties and from industry, trade unions, finance, journalism, academia, the Church, and other groups.

Strathclyde Regional Council has produced a report on the implications of unemployment for its regional services.[12] A survey of health authorities showed that almost two-thirds were doing something to respond to the health problems produced by unemployment.[13] The Archbishop of Canterbury's Commission on Urban Priority Areas made instantly controversial recommendations for improving the lot of those in the inner cities, many of which relate to unemployment.[14] The Unemployment and Health Study Group has published a report on how health services and other agencies could modify the health consequences of unemployment.[15, 16] And some district medical officers and specialists in community medicine,[17] health education departments,[18] family practitioner committees,[19] individual general practices,[20, 21] and other small but energetic groups have also set to work to try to do something for the unemployed.

The economically unsophisticated, which includes not only me and, I suspect, many doctors but also J. B. Priestley, cannot help but be struck by the contradiction of so much of Britain disintegrating at a time when so many people are unemployed. Priestley wrote in his *English Journal* in 1934: 'I think I caught a glimpse then of what may seem to future historians one of the most dreadful ironies of this time of ours, when there were never more men doing nothing and there was never so much to be done.'[22] Such ironies can be seen now very clearly in the National Health Service: many of the buildings are in a poor state of repair; waiting lists are still absurdly long; and, most important of all, many families and individuals must bear alone what can be almost impossible burdens of looking after handicapped and elderly relatives. Skilled help is of course needed to reduce waiting lists, but much of the work that cries out to be done in Britain needs only minimal skills.

Despite that, as Williams argues strongly, many of the new jobs that might be created in Britain will need considerable skills.[23] Colombo has studied where new jobs might come from in Italy, concluding that most will come from three main endeavours: new technologies and their applications; improvement of the environment and infrastructure; and human services (Table 10.1).[24] He predicts that almost two million new jobs will be created by new technology, and many of these will be highly skilled.

In one of its three models, which assumes a rapid growth in new technology, a similar but more detailed study undertaken for the

TABLE 10.1. Predictions on where new jobs will come from in Italy (Colombo)

New technologies and their applications	000's	The environment and the infrastructure	000's	Human services	000's
Robot technicians	200	Energy technicians	2–300	Medical technicians	150
New materials	200	Housing rehabilitation	150	Geriatric social workers	100
Biotechnologists	200	Hazardous waste	100	Childcare	150
Computer-aided design/ computer-aided graphics	100	Industrial conversion	150	Leisure	
Computer-aided manufacturing	100	Land rehabilitation	40		
Computer technology	450				
Testing techniques	100				
New manufacturing	300				
Office automation	300				
Total	1950	Total	640–740	Total	450

United States also predicts a huge expansion in jobs for professionally qualified people—perhaps by as much as 14 million by 2000.[25] At the same time there will be a modest increase in maintenance workers and a dramatic fall in clerical workers. These predictions assume that education and training can keep up and supply workers with the necessary skills: if they can't, then increased structural unemployment will be the result. Sadly, a report prepared jointly by the National and Economic Development Office and the Manpower Services Commission in May 1984 concluded that vocational education and training in Britain were deficient compared with that available in its three main competitors—the United States, Japan, and West Germany.[26] British companies spend only about 0.15 per cent of their turnover on training compared with 1–2 per cent in other countries.[27]

These patterns of expansion in jobs are not all prediction because they have happened to a large extent in the United States and to a much smaller extent in Britain (Table 10.2).[23, 27] In the United States between 1972 and 1982 a million jobs were lost in manufacturing industry, while the labour force increased by 23 million men and women. Unemployment did not rocket, although it did increase, because 17 million new jobs were created—mostly in the white collar sector. Over 5 million jobs were created in professional and technical occupations and 3.5 million in management and executive posts: these included 200 000 more doctors, 300 000 more computer specialists, 250 000 more lawyers, 500 000 technicians, and 150 000 social scientists. In addition, 1.3 million jobs were created in medical services at a lower level. In Britain the only sections that produced new jobs between 1979 and 1983 were health (291 000), education (120 000), business services (106 000), banking and finance (150 000), and catering (55 000). The message is thus that new jobs can appear but the conditions have to be right, and in Britain they may not be right. A very recent report from the Labour Research Group describes how the sun may already be setting on Britain's 'sunrise' industries: 'far from guaranteeing jobs and prosperity to offset the decline of other industries, the electronics industry in Britain is facing its own deep crisis.'[28]

How much the government can do to create the right conditions and new jobs is a moot point. The present British government argues that it is not for it to increase jobs but rather to create an

TABLE 10.2. Job gains and losses in Britain between June 1984 and June 1985

Sector	Numerical change (June 1984 to June 1985)	Per cent change
Services:		
Banking, finance, insurance	+79 000	+4.3
Retail distribution	+57 000	+2.7
Hotels, catering	+41 000	+4.1
Other services (public, personnel)	+24 000	+1.8
Wholesale distribution	+23 000	+2.0
Medical, other health services	+22 000	+1.7
Transport	−19 000	−2.2
Manufacturing:		
Paper, paper production, printing, publishing	+5 000	+1.0
Mechanical engineering	+3 000	+0.4
Office machines, electrical engineering, and instruments	+2 000	+0.2
Metal goods (miscellaneous)	+2 000	+0.5
Motor vehicles, parts	−9 000	−3.1
Timber, wooden furniture	−10 000	−2.2
Textiles, leather footwear, clothing	−11 000	−2.1
Other transport equipment	−13 000	−4.4
Construction	−34 000	−3.5
Coal, oil, etc.	−17 000	−5.9
Electricity, gas, water	−6 000	−1.8
Agriculture	−2 000	−0.5

environment in which businesses can produce new jobs. Others argue that the government could do more and yet don't chose to make reducing unemployment a priority. The distinguished Cambridge economist, Sir Austin Robinson, brings a long perspective to this controversy. In an essay looking back over the economics of this century he quotes his own review from 1936 of John Maynard Keynes's book, *General Theory of Employment, Interest, and Money*— 'the book that has had more effect on economic ideas than any other published in this century.'[29] In 1936 Robinson wrote:

If we accept Mr Keynes's analysis one's attitudes to many of the problems of economic policy must be substantially modified. For in a fundamental sense, and not merely in detail, the economic system, if left to itself, is not inherently stable. There is no automatic tendency to re-establish full employment in conditions of unemployment. Governments and currency authorities have a responsibility far greater than that of merely making the rules and holding the ring.

In 1986 he adds:

Economics was never the same again. One can be a monetarist and think that the restriction of the money supply will in some unexplained way prevent inflation. One may believe that wage bargains can be influenced by the level of employment. But nobody can escape the fact that you and I have a responsibility.

The evidence that unemployment harms health thus takes on great importance because the harder the evidence becomes the more difficulty the government will experience in making reducing unemployment a lower priority than reducing inflation. Williams has written:

Economic ideology has been adhered to in Britain . . . without any consciousness of the cost unemployment levies in human self respect. Perhaps there will not be enough work by the end of the century to provide everyone with a full time job, in which case hours will have to be cut and work shared out. But we are nowhere near running out of work in the mid 1980s. It is the political will to make employment the top domestic priority that is lacking.[23]

As a response to this kind of thinking a group called Charter for Jobs was formed in 1985 to lobby the government to create new jobs.[30] It has representatives from all the major political parties and from industry, trade unions, finance, journalism, academia, the Church, and other groups. Its charter is shown in the box on p. 144, but its proposals for increasing employment include: a substantial rise in public infrastructure investment with an emphasis on labour-intensive projects (which might include building the cross-channel link except that it is not very labour intensive); a cut in employer's national insurance contributions to reduce the cost of labour (without reducing wages); and a form of job guarantee for the 1.25 million long-term unemployed on projects such as those provided by the community programme.[31] The House of Commons Employment Committee has supported the idea of a job guarantee for the long-term unemployed.[32]

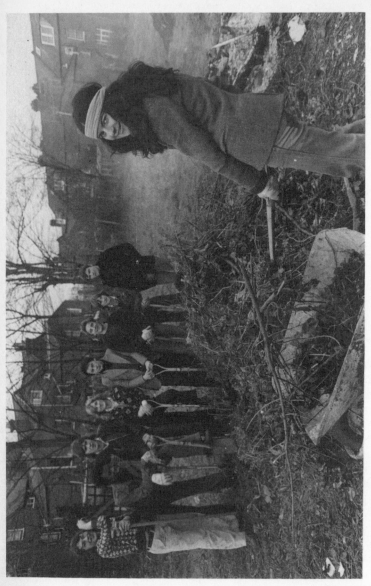

PLATE 10.1 Unemployed young people reclaim land to be used as allotments on a scheme set up by Haringey Council (picture by S. O'Meara, copyright Hulton Picture Library).

This last proposal will particularly interest those concerned about the health of the unemployed because it is the long-term unemployed and their families who suffer the most: any initiative to help them will do the most to reduce the overall harm to health. (Programmes to help them are also, as the government recognizes, the ones least likely to fuel inflation.) The Charter for Jobs wants these long-term unemployed to be offered work on socially useful projects on which they would gain work experience and be paid an hourly rate. It calculates that for an investment of £1 billion the government could provide half a million jobs, while if the money was spent in more traditional ways it would create only 100 000 jobs.

The Trades Union Congress wants to see job creation through public investment of more than £7.5 billion over the next five years: £3 billion would be spent on housing, roads, schools, and hospitals; £900 million on expanding research and development, spreading technology, and boosting exports; and £2010 million on education and the National Health Service.[33]

The *Economist* magazine has published 'a menu for the jobless' that overlaps to some extent with the ideas of the Charter for Jobs.[34] It advocates: reducing the cost of employing the least employable by cutting national insurance contributions of employers (and perhaps employees) in the hardest hit areas and perhaps for those under 25; targetting spending on those longest out of work by creating public works in inner cities and adopting labour intensity as a main criterion (as the *Economist* says, 'nothing mops up unskilled, middle aged, unemployed men like building'); and putting more effort into making areas of high unemployment attractive places in which to live and work.

The Church of England and the Confederation of British Industry are also enthusiastic about creating jobs by spending public money on building and repairing.[14] The Church, too, argues for more expenditure on public services including the National Health Service. It is upset by talk of 'proper jobs' (those that are supposed to create wealth as opposed to those that simply employ people doing useful service work) and says in its report *Faith in the City*: 'We must confront that implications for society of a belief that the manufacture of rubber ducks for export increases economic welfare, but job-creating public expenditure on environmental improvement or caring for the elderly does not.'

Many of these groups have been most concerned about the long-term unemployed, and Ashby has very ably and succinctly summarized the various policies open to the government.[35] The first is economic expansion: creating employment would become the overriding priority of the government's economic and social policies. The community programme would be expanded and positive action would be taken to ensure that those leaving the programme got the new jobs. Education and training opportunities for long-term unemployed people would also be expanded. A second option would be to take positive action—for instance, subsidies to employers—to ensure that more long-term unemployed people got jobs. If the number of jobs were not expanded, this might simply mean that long-term unemployment was shared out more.

A third policy would be to guarantee some sort of opportunity (some sort of education, training, temporary employment, work experience, or community service) to all long-term unemployed people and on taking up such an opportunity they would be paid a weekly credit on top of their supplementary benefit. The idea of the credit is that it would motivate as well as reducing the poverty associated with long-term unemployment. This is a different policy from simply increasing benefits. Although all long-term unemployed people would be offered an opportunity, it would not be compulsory and people would be free to move easily from one opportunity to another. Ashby forsees many objections to this scheme—one being that it might be regarded as 'antiwork'—and his fourth proposal is for a two-tier system. One tier would be aiming to place long-term unemployed people in employment, would offer employment and training for up to a year, and would pay the rate for the job. The second tier would offer the range of opportunities offered in the third policy option to all long-term unemployed people, and they would be paid a credit on top of their benefit for taking the opportunity. People would be able to stay in this scheme indefinitely.

These last two policies might sound rather radical, but many who have studied the future of employment would agree that radical measures are needed. Indeed, the disappearance of most employment as we know it is going to force even more radical changes. Handy in his book envisages four possible futures—derived from the work of Watts.[36]

The first future is an unemployment future in which the number of unemployed steadily increases and the gap between rich and poor widens. Those who are unemployed are not seen or heard, and those employed convince themselves that it will not happen to them, that unemployment is not that bad, and that the unemployed could get a job if they really wanted. The employed also have to bear the enormous costs of supporting the unemployed and their families or have to accede to government policies that squeeze the unemployed harder and harder. We are some way down this road, and at the end of it is a very divided society. That the disadvantaged and disenfranchized would eventually rise up and slaughter the employed in their beds is unlikely, but violence and crime would almost certainly prosper.

A second future is a one in which a small elite, aided by machines, work to produce all that is needed while the masses 'enjoy' leisure. This is Rome or Greece turned upside down, in so far as the leisured class are the least educated and skilled. Such a future is probably unworkable, not only because the economics wouldn't work, but also because such mass leisure would not provide those psychological and social necessities that most people now get from employment.

A third future is an employment future in which jobs are created regardless of whether there is enough money to pay for it all and whether there is enough work to do. The Japanese are said to have 2.5 million people in 'seatwarming' jobs and the Russians have millions in the army. The snags with this future are again the economics, but also the devaluation of employment to the point where it no longer fulfills psychological and social needs.

A fourth future is a work future in which the divisions between employment and work are broken down. Everybody would be paid a basic income (also called a social or citizen's wage) and then be free to top up his or her income with paid work. The flexibility that is coming into the labour market with new technology would then be seen not as a threat but as a boon: people could be paid work for a couple of hours a week when the children were asleep; young people could do paid work intensively when they came back from a tour round the world and before they had children, when they could slacken off while concentrating on their young. All sorts of patterns could be possible, but it would require a change in attitudes to work and employment. Attitudes are likely to change not because of advertising campaigns on television but because economic and technological changes force them.

In such a future people would not be writing books on the harmful effects of unemployment because unemployment would have no meaning. Unemployment would be gone and so would the poverty, misery, and sickness.

References

1. Handy, C. *The future of work*. Oxford: Basil Blackwell, 1985.

2. Sherman, B. *Working at leisure*. London: Methuen, 1986.

3. Robertson, J. *Future work*. Aldershot: Gower, 1985.

4. Ekins, P., ed. *The living economy. A new economics in the making*. London: Routledge and Kegan Paul, 1986.

5. Abrams, G.D., Timms, N., eds. *Values and social change in Britain*. London: Macmillan, 1985.

6. Gorz, A. *Paths to paradise: on the liberation from work*. London: Pluto Press, 1985. (French edition 1983.)

7. Holland, G. Quoted in: Felton, D. The politics of unemployment: 3. Scheme to tackle long term jobs crisis. *The Times* 1986; January 2: 4.

8. Westcott, G., Svensson, P.G., Zollner, H.F.K., eds. *Health policy implications of unemployment*. Copenhagen: World Health Organization Regional Office for Europe, 1985.

9. World Health Organization Regional Office for Europe. *Targets for health for all*. Copenhagen: WHO, 1985.

10. Janlert, U., Dahlgren, G. *Unemployment, health, and the labour market—some aspects of public health policy*. Stockholm: Swedish Health Service, 1983.

11. Balloch, S., Hume, C., Jones, B., Westland, P. *Caring for unemployed people*. London: Bedford Square Press, 1985.

12. Anonymous. *Unemployment—implications for regional services*. Glasgow: Strathclyde Regional Council, 1985.

13. Harris, C., Smith, R. What are health authorities doing about unemployment and health? *Br. Med. J.* 1987; **294**: 1076-9.

14. Archbishop of Canterbury's Commission on Urban Priority Areas. *Faith in the city: a call for action by church and nation*. London: Church House Publishing, 1985.

15. Unemployment and Health Study Group. *Unemployment, health and social policy*. Leeds: Nuffield Centre for Health Service Studies, 1984.

16. Centre for Professional Development. *Unemployment: a challenge to public health*. Manchester: Department of Community Medicine, University of Manchester, 1986.

17. Watkins, S.J. *Six aspects of the relationship between economic activity and health*. London: Faculty of Community Medicine of the Royal Colleges, 1984. (Dissertation for MFCM thesis.)

18. Black, D., Laughlin, S., eds. *Unemployment and health: resources, information, action, discussion*. Glasgow: Greater Glasgow Health Board Health Education Department, 1985. (For information and copies contact authors, Health Education Department, Greater Glasgow Health Board, 225 Bath Street, Glasgow.)

19. Kirby, J. GPs help train young jobless. *Medeconomics* 1983; December: 49–51.

20. Jarman, B. Giving advice about welfare benefits in general practice. *Br. Med. J.* 1985; **290**: 522–24.

21. Law, J. Take on staff at no cost. *Medeconomics* 1982; December: 47–51.

22. Priestley, J.B. *English journey*. Harmondsworth: Penguin, 1977.

23. Williams, S. *A job to live: the impact of tomorrow's technology on work and society*. Harmondsworth: Penguin, 1985.

24. Colombo, U. Quoted in: Williams, S. *A job to live: the impact of tomorrow's technology on work and society*. Harmondsworth: Penguin, 1985.

25. Leontief, W., Duchin, F. *The future impacts of automation on workers*. New York: Oxford University Press, 1986.

26. National Economic Development Council Manpower Services Commission: *Competence and competition*. London: NEDO, 1984.

27. Felton, D. The politics of unemployment: 2. 'Let enterprise flourish' is ministerial aim. *The Times* 1985; December 31: 2. Macintyre, D. The politics of unemployment: 5. Value of service sector jobs disputed. *The Times* 1986; January 4:2.

28. Anonymous. Sun sets on sunrise industry. *Labour Res.* 1985; **74**: 307–9.

29. Robinson, A. A child of the times. *Economist* 1986; December: 39–42.

30. Charter for Jobs. *We can cut unemployment*. London: Charter for Jobs, 1985. (PO Box 474, London NW3 4SZ.)

31. Jackman, R. *A job guarantee for long term unemployed people*. London: Employment Institute, 1986.

32. House of Commons Employment Committee. *Special employment measures and the long term unemployed.* London: HMSO, 1986.

33. Macintyre, D. The politics of unemployment: 1. Young settles in with a clear brief from Thatcher. *The Times* 1985; December 30:2.

34. Anonymous. A menu for the jobless. *Economist* 1985; December 7: 20.

35. Ashby, P. *The long term unemployed: action for a forgotten million.* London: Bedford Square Press/National Council for Voluntary Organisations, 1985.

36. Watts, A.G. *Education, unemployment and the future of work.* Milton Keynes: Open University, 1983.

11

Training and 'work' for the unemployed

MUCH is already being done to try to provide work and training for the unemployed, particularly the young unemployed, but the various programmes run by the Manpower Services Commission are not nearly as well known as they should be.[1, 2] In their survey of social workers, health visitors, and health education officers in Scotland and the Midlands in 1984, Popay *et al.* found that knowledge of local initiatives funded by the Manpower Services Commission (the MSC) was very limited, especially among health professionals.[3] Yet the commission is in its second decade and in 1984-5 was operating 4000 youth training schemes for almost 400 000 youngsters as well as running many other programmes.[1] Since then the Youth Training Scheme has been lengthened to two years, and the aim is to offer it to all 16- and 17-year-olds.[2] Harris and Smith's survey at the end of 1986 showed that health authorities had begun to pay more attention to the commission's schemes.[4]

The aims of the MSC are to 'promote a more efficient labour market and competitive workforce' and to 'help those at disadvantage in the labour market to overcome their employment problems'. The Youth Training Scheme is the largest single item in its budget, absorbing £870 million in grants in 1985-6. The rhetoric of the scheme is that it is not a way of reducing youth unemployment but rather of 'providing a permanent bridge between school and work'. If this is its aim then it is not doing awfully well because in October 1985 only 48 per cent of those emerging from the scheme were entering full-time or part-time work; a few were returning to full-time education, and 9 per cent were starting another Youth Training Scheme, but 38 per cent were going straight on to the dole.[5] Generally as youth unemployment has risen the proportion of those emerging from the scheme and finding jobs has fallen.

The scheme aims at providing not only work experience but also training, and it is intended that some of the entrants to the scheme will already be in employment. In 1984–5 about 60 per cent of 16- and 17-year-old school leavers started on the scheme, which was rather less than expected. This was because more school leavers got jobs than had been predicted, more stayed at school, and 20 000 youngsters opted not to join the scheme. (Some young people are hostile to these schemes, labelling them slave labour—the training allowance has been £27.30 but is being raised to £35 a week.) There are three strands to the scheme and each currently is supposed to last for a year: mode A caters for the unemployed and employed, is led by employers, and offers work experience to 305 000 young people in 1985–6; mode B1 is only for the unemployed, and last year offered experience with voluntary organizations, local authorities, and private sector sponsors for 80 300 young people; and mode B2 caters for the unemployed and has put 13 400 young people into schemes run by 'linked providers', largely colleges of further education and employers.

The Youth Opportunities Programme got something of a bad name for often failing to supply training or useful experience, and the Youth Training Scheme is an attempt to mend these deficiencies. Evaluation is difficult, but the quality is widely agreed to be patchy. Hearst argued that little serious evaluation had been attempted: 'Most training managers think that just to get trainees into jobs is an achievement. No attempt is being made to find out what jobs, how long their ex-trainees stay, and whether they are still being trained by their employer.'[5] Furthermore, most trainees stayed only 35 weeks on average on their year-long scheme. Yet the government has made money available to increase the programme to a two-year scheme, and costs will rise eventually to £1.1 billion.

The Archbishop of Canterbury's commission on urban priority areas confirmed its strong support both for the Manpower Services Commission in general and for the Youth Training Scheme in particular.[6] It was long overdue, the commission thought, that the effective age of starting work in Britain became 18, which is what the two-year training scheme will mean. But the MSC was disappointed that so few of those who emerged from the scheme got jobs, and it received evidence that the proportion was even lower in inner cities. Evidence was also given that black young people had great difficulty in getting on to mode A schemes.

As well as increasing funding of the Youth Training Scheme the government has also made more money available for the community programme, which is the main scheme operated by the Manpower Services Commission for helping the long-term unemployed. Temporary employment is offered on 'projects of community benefit that would not otherwise be done', and participants are paid 'a going rate' for the job. But as the commission is allowed to pay only about £67 a week for an ordinary worker this means that 72 per cent of the jobs are part time. It also means that young single people are more likely than people with families to join the scheme, and the Archbishop of Canterbury's commission wanted the pay limits relaxed for those with families.[6] The scheme is open to those who have been unemployed for the past two months and—for those aged 18-24—six of the past nine months, and—for those aged over 25-12 of the past 15 months. Since October 1984 applicants must also be in receipt directly or indirectly of a state benefit, which reduces the range of those eligible, and in particular makes it difficult for women to join. Both the Manpower Services Commission itself and the Archbishop of Canterbury's commission wanted the eligibility rules changed.

In 1984-5 about 161 000 people participated in the programme, about 12 per cent of those who have been unemployed for more than a year. In June 1985 the programme was expanded, and the plan was to reach 255 000 places by November 1986. A follow-up, which not surprisingly was uncontrolled, showed that eight months after leaving the programme about a third were employed and 5 per cent were in training.[1] A later study by a joint team from the Department of Employment and the commission made 53 recommendations on improving the programme and suggested that more attention be focused on the quality of jobs provided and the work done.[2] The commission hopes to improve the quality of the programme and in particular to increase the amount of training that participants receive.

The Archbishop of Canterbury's commission favoured the community programme but wanted it expanded.[6] It also heard many criticisms, particularly of how shattering it is to be thrown back on to the dole after a year on the programme. Many people also complained to the MSC that the training component of the programme was inadequate. Finally, the MSC thought that the programme should give priority to social services and improving inner city housing. The commission also pointed out that although the programme might help with the non-financial miseries of unemployment it does nothing for the overwhelmingly important financial aspect.

The Manpower Services Commission has for some years been running three other schemes specifically for the unemployed (see Table 11.1), and all four schemes together helped about 305 000 people in 1985-6, about 9 per cent of the unemployed. The enterprise allowance scheme helps unemployed people start their own businesses (by providing an allowance of £40 a week for up to 52 weeks), and demand has been high—about 60 000 people, almost a quarter of whom were women, were helped in 1985-6. The scheme is now being expanded. Research by the commission has shown that for every 100 businesses set up 99 jobs are created, and of the first 500 people who took advantage of the full 12-month allowance 60 per cent were still trading three years later.[7] And for every 100 businesses still trading after two years an additional 99 full and part time jobs had been created.[2]

The voluntary projects programme allows unemployed people to undertake voluntary work without their state benefits being affected, and the community industry scheme helps young people who are 'personally or socially disadvantaged' by providing up to a year of work of benefit to the community.

The commission has also started some new initiatives for the long-term unemployed. In January 1986 the commission began offering long-term unemployed people in nine areas in-depth counselling at a Job Centre, a week-long Restart course designed to give participants a more 'positive' approach, and a Job Start allowance for those who took lower paid jobs. In March 1986 the Chancellor extended these pilot schemes to the whole country, and the aim is to interview all the long-term unemployed by March 1987. The government was claiming in November 1986 that through Restart one in five of the long-term unemployed had left the register. Between 12 May and 9 October 336 451 people were interviewed and 2547 (0.8 per cent) were placed in jobs, 9757 (2.9 per cent) on the community programme, 2508 (0.7 per cent) to job clubs, 1585 (0.5 per cent) to the Enterprise Allowance Scheme, 5488 (1.6 per cent) to training, 31 012 (9.2 per cent) to Restart courses, and 1054 (0.3 per cent) to the voluntary projects programme. What the government has not said is that in the same quarter of last year—before Restart began— 18.7 per cent of the long-term unemployed left the register. Nevertheless, the government plans to extend the scheme to those who have been unemployed for only six months.

Job clubs are a slightly older initiative where long-term unemployed people can meet and help each other to find work. Thirty people meet for three hours four days a week and must apply for at least 10 jobs each day. Pilot schemes have shown that 70 per cent of the members of the clubs find work, and the commission is now aiming at increasing the number of clubs to 450.

Many of these schemes were not, until very recently, nearly as well known as they should have been, and certainly health authorities and doctors did not seem to know much about them, although there had been isolated examples of health authorities,[8, 9] general practitioners,[10] and family practitioner committees[11] taking on people through the schemes. Now things may be improving.[4] The National Health Service is the biggest employer in Western Europe and is still far from meeting all health needs; yet in 1985 only 0.5 per cent of places on the community programme were taken up by health authorities, compared with 45 per cent by local authorities—and 60 per cent of the NHS take up was by four Merseyside authorities. Victor Paige, who was the chairman of the NHS management board (and previously a Manpower Services commissioner), wrote to all regional health authority chairmen drawing attention to the low take up.

The Health Services Management Unit at Manchester University has conducted some research into why the uptake was so slow. The problems seemed to be resistance from trade unions, although these are often the same unions as have co-operated with local authorities; authorities thinking that they do not have the managers spare to supervise the schemes; a general preoccupation with the implementation of the Griffiths plan for reorganization may have kept administrators' minds on other matters; and, which may be the main reason, the fact that few individual managers have had any commitment to such schemes.

Harris and Smith in their survey also found that trade union resistance was often mentioned as a reason for not taking on more people through the commission's schemes, but the general manager

TABLE 11.1. Characteristics of selected Manpower Services Commission programmes

Programme	Youth training scheme	Community programme	Enterprise allowance scheme	Voluntary projects programme
Places in 1984-5	389 400	132 800	46 000	280 projects (63 000 volunteers)
Cost 1984-5 (£m)	849.5	534.3	80.1	9.9
Available to	All 16-year-old school leavers Unemployed 17-year-old leavers All disabled under 21	Unemployed for previous two months plus (if between 18 and 24) at least six of last nine months or (if 25 or over) 12 of the last 15 months; must be in receipt of state benefit	Unemployed for 13 weeks or under notice of redundancy for 13 weeks; must have £1000 (usually easily borrowed)	Unemployed people

Duration	One year	One year	One year	One year
Work and training provided	Work and training with private employers, voluntary organizations, local authorities, colleges of further education. Includes 13 weeks 'off the job' training	Work on 'projects of community benefit that would otherwise not be done'	Allowance of up to £40 a week to start own business	Work on voluntary projects that bring new skills and develop old ones
Payment	£27.30	Up to £60.00 per week		No payment, but state benefits not affected
'Results'	48 per cent get full- or part-time work; 9 per cent start another scheme; 38 per cent back into unemployment	40 per cent find a job in the next 12 months	100 businesses create 50 extra jobs; 60 per cent of businesses still trading after three years	
Planned expansion	Scheme being increased to two years; cost up to £1.1 billion	To 230 000 places by June 1986; cost £711m	Places being increased to 80 000; period of qualification reduced to 8 weeks	Budget being increased to £12 m; greater emphasis to be placed on education, training, and community work

of the south-east unit of Northumberland District Health Authoity expressed well some other difficulties:

The main problems are that we have to pay the going rate for the job and the MSC will reimburse only to £67 a week and that the work undertaken must not be that which would normally be done by employees of the organisation. This in particular is very difficult to match because we therefore have to look for special projects. The old work experience schemes used to allow us to employ individuals to actually learn skills such as gardening or clerical or typing work.[4]

When the finances of the authorities are so tightly stretched they are unwilling to take on any extra expenditure and are also not keen to fund projects that are not absolutely essential. But, by taking on more people under the many schemes operated by the commission, health authorities and individual doctors could not only get more done but could also help raise the health and morale of those that the authorities take on—and their families.

An excellent example of what can be done comes from South Sefton Health Authority, where more than 250 long-term unemployed people are being used to staff a large health promotion programme, give dental education,[8, 9] undertake a community survey of health behaviour, provide a day and night sitting service, and maintain security in the authority hospitals. This considerable scheme (almost certainly the largest in the NHS) has grown up over five years and has needed careful and intensive management. It is now serving as an inspiration to start other such schemes, and Dr Hilary Hodge, the dentist who started it all, believes that the main impediment to there being more such schemes is a professional attitude that does not accept that long-term unemployed people can manage such work. Dr Hodge has, however, produced controlled evaluations of her original dental health education schemes which show that they have worked.[12]

Dr Hodge began the scheme in a small way five years ago when she arrived in South Sefton with the responsibility for developing dental health and found that she had few staff and resources. As she says, 'You need people to educate other people.' So she looked around and came across the Manpower Service Commission's Youth Opportunities Programme. She took on 10 young people, many of whom were alienated, low achievers, and depressed, and had low self-esteem. With careful and gentle supervision these young people were turned into health workers. Their first exposure was to children in a preschool playgroup, and with them they gained confidence.

Next Dr Hodge took on 11 long-term unemployed adults, many of whom were teachers and other professionals, and with them she produced dental health education packages. These were developed, implemented, and tested, and are now used by other health authorities. About 40 per cent of those who worked on the scheme subsequently got jobs, and eight have gone on to train as health education officers. It was two years ago, still under the supervision of Dr Hodge, that the range of services provided by these unemployed people expanded, and in the last few months many other health authorities have become interested. Dr Hodge emphasizes the importance of starting small and working hard with the participants and their supervisors because things can go wrong. The participants' motivation must be maintained, or they begin to think that they are being fobbed off with jobs 'that are not proper jobs'.

Another exciting project is one that uses 120 people from the community programme to produce art for hospitals and residential homes of Tower Hamlets and Hackney.[13] Those on the project also create gardens for the disabled, produce health education material, and work with long-term patients. More than 60 per cent go on to get jobs afterwards.

The real beauty of these projects is that they have helped not only the unemployed but also the employed of South Sefton and East London. Other health authorities have developed schemes—for instance, Haringey Health Authority has used unemployed people as interpreters—and so have some family practitioner committees and even some individual general practitioners. Redbridge and Waltham Forest Family Practitioner Committee took people on the youth training scheme and trained them as receptionists,[10] and some individual general practitioners have also trained unemployed young people as receptionists.[11]

Together with the Health Education Council, Dr Hodge and others from South Sefton have produced a guide on how health authorities and individuals can use the Manpower Services Commission community programme.[14] *Medeconomics* has already published a guide for doctors on how to use the commission,[11] but

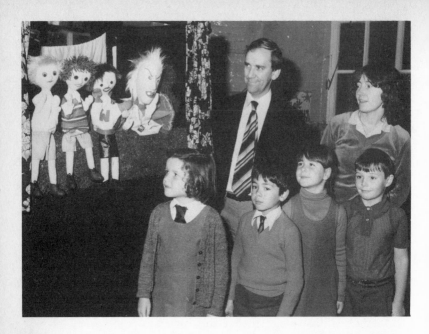

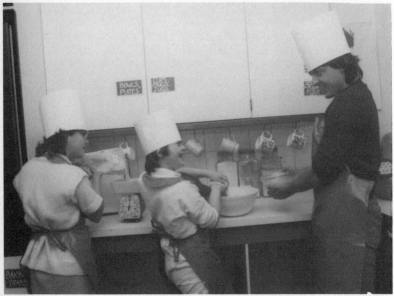

PLATE 11.1 Top: schoolchildren watch a puppet show used in the South Sefton dental health education programme created by unemployed people on the community programme (copyright Sefton Newspapers Ltd). Below: an unemployed man on the community programme works with handicapped children at a Scottish adventure playground (MSC Crown copyright).

any health worker interested should be able to get help from his or her local job centre.

As well as creating new 'jobs', employers have a part to play in sharing out the employment that is available. Working days, weeks, years, and lives are becoming progressively shorter, but these changes have not been associated with any widespread increase in sharing out the paid employment available. Too often reduced working weeks, rotating periods of worklessness, and early retirement have occurred in industries that are hard pressed, and, as the Unemployment and Health Study Group says, have been a means for sharing out miseries rather than benefits.[15]

Work can be shared in a variety of ways. One possibility is for two people to do one job between them, and this is happening in many sectors—including health. Often it is married women with children who share, but GEC, concerned by high unemployment among young people around its plants, offered split-starter jobs.[16] The new recruits worked half time and received half wages, and spent the rest of their time in voluntary training or further education. If one partner was ill or on holiday then the other would work full time, meaning that the employers could always be sure of somebody to do the job. When, as happened, the industry picked up, the half timers became full timers, which again was advantageous to the employers because they had trained people available immediately.

Sabbaticals are a second way of sharing work, and although familiar to some academics are almost unknown in the rest of Britain. They, too, might benefit both employee and employer if intelligently used, because often those on sabbaticals will use the time to learn new skills at a time when many are finding their traditional skills inadequate for their changing jobs. Shorter working weeks and working days are likely to benefit the health of the employed and their families as well as that of the unemployed and their families if the work goes to the unemployed. The same applies to longer holidays. Early retirement is a phrase that strikes terror into some because it has too often been a way of concentrating unemployment among psychologically and financially unprepared older workers. But it need not be like that.

All of these trends could be encouraged by governments making grants to support job sharing, legislating to limit working hours and guarantee longer holidays and a right to part-time work, and adjusting pension rules so that it was easier to take sabbaticals and retire early in financial security.[17] Such measures would need to be accompanied, Watkins argues, with measures to increase leisure possibilities—for example, support for sports facilities, education programmes, and increased rights of access to the countryside.

Organizations and individuals can thus do a great deal to reduce the misery of unemployment by pointing unemployed people towards these many schemes and by using them on projects of their own. Health workers may not think that it is any part of their job to help find work for the unemployed, but when the evidence is so strong that unemployment harms health it seems to me that it should be. And the most exciting thing of all is that the unemployed can be used on projects to help raise health standards. A glance through two issues of *Community Programme News* shows all sorts of imaginative projects related to health:[18, 19] unemployed people are being used in health education, to help mentally handicapped children and other disabled people, to improve communications for the deaf, to man a help line, and in campaigns against hypothermia.

References

1. Manpower Services Commission. *Annual report 1984–1985*. Sheffield: MSC, 1985.

2. Manpower Services Commission. *Annual report 1985–1986*. Sheffield: MSC, 1986.

3. Popay, J., Dhooge, Y., Shipman, C. *Unemployment and health: what role for health and social services?* London: Department of Social Sciences, Polytechnic of the Southbank, 1985.

4. Harris, C., Smith, R. What are health authorities doing about unemployment and health? *Br. Med. J.* 1987; **294**: 1076–9.

5. Hearst, D. A teenage revolution that failed at work. *Guardian* 1985; July 3: 11.

6. Archbishop of Canterbury's Commission on Urban Priority Areas. *Faith in the city: a call for action by church and nation*. London: Church House Publishing, 1985.

7. Felton, D. The politics of unemployment: 2. 'Let enterprise flourish' is ministerial aim. *The Times*; 1986 December 31: 2.

8. Hodge, H. Manpower for dental health. *Health & Social Serv. J.* 1985; May 30: 676–7.

9. Hodge, H., Griffiths, B.B. Dental health education and the Manpower Services Commission youth training scheme. *Health Educ. J.* 1985; **44**: 124-7.

10. Law, J. Take on staff at no cost. *Medeconomics* 1982; December: 47-51.

11. Kirby, J. GPs help train young jobless. *Medeconomics* 1983; December: 49-51.

12. Hodge, H., Buchanan, M., Jones, J., O'Donnell, P. The evaluation of the infant dental health education programme developed in Sefton. *Community Dental Health J.* 1985; **2**: 175-85.

13. Smith, R. Beauty and the dole. *Br. Med. J.* 1986; **293**: 1632-35.

14. McVey, D., Barnett, C., Hodge, H. *Guide to the MSC community programme*. Liverpool: South Sefton Health Authority, 1986.

15. Unemployment and Health Study Group. *Unemployment, health and social policy*. Leeds: Nuffield Centre for Health Service Studies, 1984.

16. Williams, S. *A job to live: the impact of tomorrow's technology on work and society*. Harmondsworth: Penguin, 1985.

17. Watkins, S.J. Recession and health—the policy implications. In: Westcott, G., Svensson, P.G., Zollner, H.F.K., eds. *Health policy implications of unemployment*. Copenhagen: World Health Organization Regional Office for Europe, 1985.

18. *Community Programme News* 1985; November.

19. *Community Programme News* 1986; January.

12

Financial and local action to help the unemployed

MOST unemployed people, and particularly those with families, have incomes much lower than when they were working, and many slide into poverty.[1, 2, 3] More than anything else poverty may be the link between unemployment and poor health;[4] so raising the living standards of the unemployed may be one of the most effective ways of improving their health. This can be achieved by increasing benefits and their uptake and by reducing the price of travel, entertainment, educational facilities, and the like for the unemployed. The Archbishop of Canterbury's commission also makes the important point that how benefits are made available matters as well as how much is given.[5] At the moment the experience of claiming benefits is becoming steadily more stressful and humiliating.

The government recognizes that our outdated social security system is falling apart under the enormous strain and has embarked on what it has called 'the most fundamental examination of our social security system since the Second World War.'[6-9] The present system, it says, is too complex, fails to support those who need it most, and leaves many people trapped in poverty and unemployment. The aim of the suggested reforms is thus to simplify the system and get more benefits to those who need them most. But another important aim is to create a 'secure financial base for the social security system', and many groups are suspicious that these much trumpeted reforms are in fact a cost-cutting exercise. Critics are worried that the introduction of the reforms in April 1988 may increase the gap between the rich and the poor, a gap that has been widening steadily in Britain since the Second World War.[6]

The main proposals relevant to the unemployed are the replacement of supplementary benefit by income support and of the family income supplement by family credits; housing benefits are also to be

substantially reformed and simplified. In addition, dozens of existing
benefits will be replaced by the social fund, which will make loans
rather than grants. What will happen to unemployment benefit is
not yet clear, and a government study is now in progress 'to see what
improvements can be made to the arrangements for paying benefits
to the unemployed'.[9]

What matters most to the unemployed is whether they will have
more or less money under the new system, and this will not be
known for sure until the new system begins. But the government has
calculated that the families of the long-term unemployed will be
£1.40 a week better off under the new system. The Policy Studies Institute, however, says that the long-term unemployed with families
will be either no better off or worse off.[10] This is because they claim
that many of the single payments—for items such as furniture, bed-
ding, and cookers—are to be replaced by loans that will have to be
repaid. The Institute says that the average family claims £3.20 a
week in such payments and so will be £1.80 a week worse off. The
National Consumer Council has made similar calculations and also
concludes that unemployed families will on average be £1.60 a week
worse off.[11] This may sound like a paltry sum to those who regularly
spend this amount on a lunchtime gin and tonic, but the proposed
basic rate for unemployed couples is £48 a week; those with children
will get a family premium of £5.75.

The council also points out that under the new proposals it will
still be very difficult for the unemployed to do any casual or part
time work without losing benefit.[11] At the moment they can earn £4
without losing benefit, and under the new scheme it will be increased
to £5. If it had been uprated with inflation since 1975, the council
points out, it would now be worth £10. Another snag for the
unemployed with the new scheme is that they are likely to end up
with smaller pensions. Although the state earnings-related pension
scheme is not to be abolished—as was originally proposed—the
pension will now no longer be calculated on the best 20 years. This
means that every spell of unemployment will lead to a smaller
pension.

The Child Poverty Action Group is also concerned that the
reforms do not discuss increasing uptake. Because of the low uptake
of many means-tested benefits the group argued for increases in
universal benefits such as child benefit. The government dismissed

this approach as too expensive and also argued that too much of the money would then end up in the pockets of the well-off.

Whether or not the proposed reforms are going to slightly increase or decrease the income of long-term unemployed families, they are certainly not going to lead to the substantial increase that would be necessary to reduce the ill health of the unemployed and their families. The Archbishop of Canterbury's commission advocated a more radical package that included paying the long-term unemployed the long-term supplementary benefit rate, substantially increasing child benefit, and raising the amount that social security claimants could earn before losing benefit.[5] It also wanted a major review of the system that, unlike the government's, would be independent, consider the whole welfare system, and consider what benefits are supposed to cover—because many people think that current benefits are set far too low. The commission would also like such a review to consider the radical proposal that all people should be paid a basic income.

Dilnot, an economist at the Institute of Fiscal Studies, has costed the proposals of the Archbishop's commission, which also include doubling the Manpower Services Commission community programme, spending more on houses, sewers, and roads, increasing the rate support grant, and expanding the urban programme of inner city projects.[12] The total costs would be about £4 billion, which would mean 4p on the standard rate of income tax. To politicians of many colours this seems like a non-starter, but another way of looking at the issue is to recognize that the abolition of income tax relief on mortgages would raise £4.5 billion. Early last year an inquiry into British housing chaired by the Duke of Edinburgh advocated just such a proposal, although recognizing that it would have to be phased in over 10 years to avoid severe hardship.[13]

The Archbishop of Canterbury's commission addressed the question of whether the better-off would be willing to make financial sacrifices to alleviate the misery of the poor and unemployed, and many at least say that they would.[5] A survey in *Social Trends* showed that three-quarters of the population thought that the gap between rich and poor was too large, and a third wanted taxation increased and more spent on health and social security.[14] Only 9 per cent wanted tax cuts with less spent on health and social security. The commission says that this confirms the news that altruism is still alive in Britain, and it repeats many times the sobering figures on the widening gap between rich and poor.

In 1976 the worst-off fifth of the population received 7.4 per cent of national income, while the best-off fifth received 37.9 per cent; by 1983 the best-off fifth had increased their share to 39.6 per cent, while that of the poorest had decreased to 6.9 per cent (see Table 12.1).[15] The gap in original household income (from employment, occupational pensions, and investments, and from other households—for example, alimony, gifts, etc.—but excluding that from state pensions and benefits) is even wider: in 1983 the poorest 20 per cent had an original income of £120 while for the richest 20 per cent it was £18 640. And this inequality is widening much faster than the inequality in final income: in 1976 the poorest 20 per cent earned 0.8 per cent of original income as opposed to 44.4 per cent

TABLE 12.1. Distribution of original, disposable, and final household income

	Quintile groups of households				
	Bottom fifth	Next fifth	Middle fifth	Next fifth	Top fifth
Original income*					
1976	0.8	9.4	18.8	26.6	44.4
1981	0.6	8.1	18.0	26.9	46.4
1982	0.4	7.1	18.2	27.2	47.1
1983	0.3	6.7	17.7	27.2	48.0
Disposable income†					
1976	7.0	12.6	18.2	24.1	38.1
1981	6.7	12.1	17.7	24.1	39.4
1982	6.8	11.8	17.6	24.2	39.6
1983	6.9	11.9	17.6	24.0	39.6
Final income‡					
1976	7.4	12.7	18.0	24.0	37.9
1981	7.1	12.4	17.9	24.0	38.6
1982	6.9	12.0	17.6	24.1	39.4
1983	6.9	12.2	17.6	24.0	39.3

* Income from employment, occupational pensions, investments, and from other households—for example, alimony, gifts.
† Original income plus state benefits minus income tax and national insurance contributions.
‡ Disposable income minus indirect taxes plus imputed benefits from government expenditure on items like health and education.

for the richest 20 per cent; by 1983 the proportions were 0.3 per cent and 48 per cent.

To a small extent this staggering gap in original income between the rich and the poor is offset by state benefits, but the uptake of many of these is low. Potential recipients are unaware of benefits to which they are entitled, baffled by the complexity of the social security system, unwilling to accept 'charity', scared of the stigma attached to attending social security offices, humiliated by the experiences they have in these offices, and ignorant of the many sources of advice on benefits—Citizens Advice Bureau, etc. Doctors and other health workers could play a key part in increasing the uptake of benefits because almost everybody has a general practitioner, two-thirds of the population visit him or her at least once each year, and consulting the doctor or his practice staff carries nothing like the same stigma as attending a social security office.

Yet most general practitioners do not see it as part of their job to advise their patients on benefits, and, indeed, most know little about the rules for the roughly 30 state benefits currently available.[16] Jarman has calculated in his inner London practice that about 1427 (2.3 per cent) of 62 829 primary diagnoses made in 1979–81 were connected with social circumstances—and 565 (40 per cent) of those were related to financial problems.[17] He also looked at the patients whom he, his partners, or practice staff visited regularly, and discovered that a third were not receiving an attendance allowance to which they were entitled.

Jarman responded by writing a computer program that helped people—with the aid of an operator from the local social security office—to find out about benefits they might be entitled to. The operator holds a 'surgery' every morning in the health centre for booked and unbooked patients, and he also accepts referrals from other health practitioners. The program takes about 10 minutes to run through if people know the necessary details about themselves—for example, their weekly rent—and longer if they do not.

This project shows that general practitioners can help their patients by providing this information on benefits without having to learn for themselves the details of the social security system and without having to prolong their consultations by thumbing through manuals. Other practitioners might achieve the same result in different ways—perhaps by inviting into their health centres volunteers from the local Citizens' Advice Bureau, or perhaps by using somebody from the Manpower Services Commission community programme to operate the computer. Once the will is there and once general practitioners think that it should be part of their job to provide this information, then a service can easily be established.[17]

Providing information on benefits is also an important part of the work of local authorities that have taken the initiative in trying to improve the lot of the unemployed—as it is for the many other national and local organizations trying to do something for the unemployed. But most of these groups are also trying to do much more.

The Association of Metropolitan Authorities has urged its members to think what they can do for the unemployed,[18] and Strathclyde Regional Council has published a draft plan.[19] The thinking behind the council's plan is that everything possible must be done to create new jobs and that 'unemployment should never be accepted as a satisfactory option because its effects on people are intolerable'. But at the same time the council accepts that unemployment is likely to continue (and probably to get worse) in Strathclyde, that it can do much to lessen the impact of unemployment on communities and individuals, and that in the long term 'a solution is unlikely to be found without a fundamental change in the way society views work and how it should be rewarded'. This is progressive and practical thinking from north of the border and seems to be part of a growing tradition of confronting problems head on rather than edging round them as is so often the way in England.[20, 22]

Strathclyde Regional Council wants each of its departments to examine what they can do about unemployment, which will mean 'in-service training, secondment of staff to work with and support voluntary effort in local communities and challenging the "way we've always done it" approach to service delivery'. Each group will be required 'as a matter of urgency' to devise 'a comprehensive information service, a counselling service for unemployed people, a training package for staff, and a means of continuing direct communication links with the unemployed'. This last requirement is particularly important because so many initiatives for helping the unemployed have foundered on the fact that the unemployed tend to be scattered, alone, and unreachable.[23]

Information is to be directed firstly at those who are about to become unemployed; rarely in the past have employers made an attempt to prepare people for unemployment. Workers about to be made redundant can be helped to find other jobs, retrained, or at the very least advised about the implications of being unemployed and the many sources of help available. Although such schemes have been operated in the United States and occasionally in this country—when the Talbot plant in Linwood was threatened with closure, and when the British Steel Corporation closed the Consett steel works—they are still unusual.[24]

The other groups at whom Strathclyde Regional Council will aim information will be those already unemployed, those about to leave school, and their own staff. Information will cover financial matters, Regional and District Council services, training opportunities, alternative sources of employment, and health and community matters. The council will use the mass media as well its own staff and offices, and it is also concerned to get across to the general public 'the causes, scale, and effects of unemployment generally on individuals, families, local services, and society'. This general education is particularly important if our society is going to change its often negative attitude to the unemployed and the way that it views work.

The counselling that the council wants its staff to provide is to be 'independent, honest, flexible, persistent (when required), informal, and confidential' and will help unemployed people and their families work through their problems as well as point them towards the practical steps that they can take to alleviate their plight.

The Regional Council plan makes many other specific recommendations and includes a whole section on health. But most of the recommendations on health are decidedly vague, and encouragement of health authorities to monitor the effects of unemployment on health and devise a plan for reducing its impact has met little response. Health authorities have been even slower than most local authorities to take any action on unemployment and health. Why this should be so needs to be further explored, but it is something to do with the attitude of health authorities to the unemployed, a failure to appreciate the effects of unemployment on health, an unwillingness to accept that responding to unemployment is part of their job, and a general preoccupation with other matters such as reorganization and cuts.

I cannot begin to describe the whole range of initiatives taken by local groups, but Table 12.2 (after Popay *et al.*[24]) gives an idea of what might be available in one area. Local directories have been produced—for instance, in Lewisham, London,[25] and in Strathclyde[21]—and ideally all health workers should have access to such a directory. Producing one might be a priority for any local unemployment and health group, and useful national addresses are included in the next chapter.

Two national initiatives with local branches deserve further mention. In 1980 the Trades Union Congress launched a campaign to organize services for the unemployed and set up a network of unemployed workers' centres. There are now about 210 of these, and they vary from place to place.[26] The kinds of services they offer are shown in Table 12.3, but generally they offer advice; social, educational, and recreational facilities; jobs and training; and programmes to change public attitudes about unemployment. Another scheme is Church Action with the Unemployed, which now has a national network. Its three main activities are pastoral care, job creation, and providing work experience; Table 12.4 gives ideas on what groups might do. Many health workers, whether or not they are Christians, might find inspiration from these suggestions.

TABLE 12.2. Examples of local initiatives to help the unemployed

Advisory/communication

Careers advice office
Citizens' Advice Bureau
Claimants' union
Community resource centre
Directory of community initiatives
Financial advice centre
Law centre
Local liaison initiative
Phone-in service
Radio programme
Resource pack
Resources register
Welfare rights group

Counselling/psychological help

Alcohol centre
Community programmes
Depression group
Playbridge
Pre-redundancy counselling scheme
Youth clubs

Ethnic groups

Advice/library facilities project
Community relations council
Community work course for mature
black/white people
Multiracial community centre
Preparatory course for mature black
people
Racism awareness training unit
Training for black people in
management

Job creation

Community industry project
Community schemes to increase
employment
Disabled workshop
Employment and training project
Push to employ youngsters previously
in care

Leisure/recreation

Bussing scheme
Community centres
Leisure scheme

Leisure passport
Librarian for the unemployed
Sports centre

Retraining/education

Adult education
Careers advice
Course for mature black people
wishing to enter caring professions
Disablement retraining
Employment and training project
Handicapped social skills course
Long-term unemployed training
Retraining older workers scheme
Technical college summer project
Training programme for young/
disabled
Women's training directory
Youth Training Scheme/
Youth Opportunities Programme/
Manpower Services Commission
Youth clubs
Youth community workshop

Practical needs

Food co-operative
Furniture recycling

Women

Women and employment resources
centre
Women and social security group
Women's training directory
Young women's employment group

Youth groups

Advice and counselling projects
Detached youth project
Information and training project
Youth aid
Youth clubs
Youth leisure project
Youth project—drop in
Youth service unemployment project
Phone-in service
Special local projects
Youth inquiry service
Young Men's Christian Association

TABLE 12.3. Activities of the TUC unemployed workers' centres

Information

Materials provided by public, voluntary, and trade union bodies

Advice and counselling

'Surgeries' with local authority officials
Referral services
Legal advice

Education

Classes on adult literacy and numeracy
Courses on TUC campaigns, e.g. 'Unemployment: the fight for
    TUC alternatives'
Workshops on pottery, printing, photography
Readers groups, linked with libraries, books donated by local groups

Arts

Drama groups
'Keep fit' sessions
Discos, particularly for the young unemployed

Representation

Campaigning for free use of leisure facilities and travel
Providing meeting rooms and facilities for young people on
    Youth Opportunities Programme and union representatives
Arranging surgeries with full-time union officials and direct union
    representation before tribunals

Organization

Preparing newsletters for distribution at supplementary benefit offices
Organizing 'outreach' work to make contact with the unemployed at home
Organizing visits to workplaces and trade union branches for school
    and college leavers
Providing facilities for unemployed women's groups and
    unemployed blacks' groups

Crèche facilities

Children's books and toys
After school collection service

Cookery

Imaginative cheap meals provided at low cost

Sports

Mainly five a side football fixtures at present, for young
    unemployed

TABLE 12.4. Practical action advocated by Church Action with the Unemployed

---

Pastoral care

(Coping with being out of work)

• Start an unemployment group. Identify the special needs of unemployed people in your locality.

• Open a centre where people can meet for helpful counselling and advice.

• Adapt church premises for use as a drop-in or resource centre for action, information, leisure, and recreation.

• Join with others in setting up self-help groups.

• Promote discussion in your congregation on the changing role of work in life.

• Make unemployment the subject of a sermon or an article in your magazine.

Work experience

(A better chance to get jobs)

• Sponsor a scheme under the Manpower Services Commission (MSC) Youth Training Schemes. Provide young people with work experience on employers' premises. Set up a training workshop. Devise a project of benefit to the community. Get money and help from the MSC.

• Sponsor a scheme under the MSC Community Programme. Provide those adults who have been out of work for longer periods with temporary work of community benefit. Money and help are also available from the MSC.

• Note that these MSC special programmes do not create permanent jobs and are in a sense palliative. But they do offer training and experience which can help people, especially young people, to have a better chance of getting jobs that are available. Insist on high quality schemes that give real training.

Job creation

(New jobs and permanent work)

• Join with others to create a new job administering your new churches or maintaining the premises.

• Start a neighbourhood co-operative to do gardening and odd jobs work, to clean windows and cars, to go shopping and do housework for people.

• Start an industrial common-ownership enterprise. Join with others to use redundancy money as start-up capital.

• Start a new business using existing local resources and skills.

• Ask the Department of Industry and the MSC what loans and grants are available to finance these activities.

• Persuade employers to take on extra people.

References

1. Moylan, S., Millar, J., Davies, R. *For richer, for poorer? DHSS study of unemployed men.* London: HMSO, 1984.

2. White, M. *Long term unemployment and labour markets.* London: Policy Studies Institute, 1983.

3. Smith, R. 'Gissa job': the experience of unemployment. *Br. Med. J.* 1985; **291**: 1263–6.

4. Warr, P. Twelve questions about unemployment and health. In: Roberts, R., Finnegan, R., Gallie, D., eds. *New approaches to economic life*. Manchester: Manchester University Press, 1985.

5. Archbishop of Canterbury's Commission on Urban Priority Areas. *Faith in the city: a call for action by church and nation*. London: Church House Publishing, 1985.

6. Department of Health and Social Security. *Reform of social security*. Vol 1. London: HMSO, 1985. (Cmnd 9517).

7. Department of Health and Social Security. *Reform of social security*. Vol II. *Programme for change*. London: HMSO, 1985. (Cmnd 9518).

8. Department of Health and Social Security. *Reform of social security*. Vol III. *Background papers*. London: HMSO, 1985. (Cmnd 9519).

9. Department of Health and Social Security. *Reform of social security. Programme for action*. London: HMSO, 1985. (Cmnd 9691).

10. Timmins, N. Poorest families 'will not benefit'. *The Times* 1985; December 19: 5.

11. National Consumer Council. *The government's social security proposal. Briefing paper No 1. The long term unemployed still put at the bottom of the heap*. London: NCC, 1986.

12. Dilnot, A. Quoted in: Lipsey, D. How much would it cost? *Sunday Times* 1985; December 8: 17.

13. Bazlinton, C., ed. *Inquiry into British housing*. London: National Federation of Housing Associations, 1985.

14. Jowell, R., Airey, C. British social attitudes. In: Central Statistical Office, *Social Trends 1985*. London: HMSO, 1985.

15. Central Statistical Office. *Social Trends 1986*. London: HMSO, 1986.

16. Jarman, B. Giving advice about welfare benefits in general practice. *Br. Med. J.* 1985; **290**: 522-4.

17. Cohen, R. Personal view. *Br. Med. J.* 1986; **292**: 54.

18. Balloch, S., Hume, C., Jones, B., Westland, P. *Caring for unemployed people: a study of the impact of unemployment on demand for personal social services*. London: Bedford Square Press, 1985. (Prepared for the Association of Metropolitan Authorities.)

19. Anonymous. *Unemployment—implications for regional services*. Glasgow: Strathclyde Regional Council, 1985.

20. Black, D., Laughlin, S., eds. *Unemployment and health: resources, information, action, discussion*. Glasgow: Greater Glasgow Health Board Health Education Department, 1985. (For information and copies contact authors,

Health Education Department, Greater Glasgow Health Board, 225 Bath Street, Glasgow.)

21. Scottish Health Education Coordinating Committee. *Health education in the prevention of alcohol related problems.* Edinburgh: Scottish Home and Health Department, 1985.

22. Anonymous. Scots lead the way on alcohol. *Br. Med. J.* 1985; **290**: 952-3.

23. Popay, J. Responding to unemployment at a local level. In: Westcott, G., Svensson, P.G., Zollner, H.F.K. *Health policy implications of unemployment.* Copenhagen: World Health Organization Regional Office for Europe, 1985.

24. Popay, J., Dhooge, Y., Shipman, C. *Unemployment and health: what role for health and social services?* London: Health Education Council, 1986.

25. Voluntary Action Lewisham. *Directory of employment and training projects in Lewisham.* London: Voluntary Action Lewisham, 1985. (Address for copy: Voluntary Action Lewisham, Employment Development Unit, 120 Rushey Green, London SE6.)

26. Trades Union Congress. *TUC centres for the unemployed.* London: TUC, 1985.

13

Improving the health of the unemployed A job for health authorities and health workers

HEALTH authorities and health workers have been slow to wake up to the considerable health implications of mass unemployment. It is 15 years since British unemployment first hovered around the million mark, and more than 10 years since the rapid increase began. Even 15 years ago there was ample evidence—much of it from work done in the 1930s—that unemployment was associated with ill health and an increased workload for hospitals and general practitioners. Since then, despite much of the necessary research not having been done, the evidence that unemployment harms health and brings people to their doctors has grown much stronger.

Yet still no health authority has published a comprehensive strategy for tackling health problems caused by unemployment, and few have understood that they could themselves—as large employers—offer work opportunities to the unemployed, either on their own initiative or through the Manpower Services Commission. The departments of health have only recently and grudgingly accepted the importance of unemployment in harming health. None of the Royal Colleges has published a report on the problem, and, although the British Medical Association now has a working party looking at inequalities and health, it has not addressed itself to unemployment.

One group that has recognized the importance of the issue is the Health Visitors Association, which held a week long meeting on unemployment more than five years ago. Finally, although some individual doctors and other health workers grasped the implications of unemployment for health long ago,[1] most did not and still have not.

Popay *et al.* studied 40 health visitors, 19 health education officers, and 51 social workers in three regions—London, the Midlands, and Scotland—to see how unemployment was affecting their work, to discover how they were responding, and to explore why much of the response had been *ad hoc* and inadequate.[2] More than 80 per cent of health visitors and social workers thought that unemployment was affecting their day-to-day practice, but only about half of the health education officers thought so. The increase in poverty was what had hit most of the practitioners, but the health visitors and social workers also found that they were having to manage individual and family problems that were created, exacerbated, and made much more complex by unemployment.

Despite recognizing that unemployment was affecting their work, most were ignorant of many of the local initiatives being taken to help unemployed people and most were responding in a purely *ad hoc* way. Very few had stopped to consider whether what they were doing was the best way of responding. The poor response resulted partly from a lack of time and resources, but there were other reasons: an attitude that unemployment and its effects were not matters for health or social work professionals; thoughts by health professionals that it was a matter for other professionals, particularly social workers; confusion about what could be done and a lack of conviction that anything was effective; ideas that the way that their training and work patterns made them respond was the wrong way; worries that they could only ameliorate and not remove the difficulties; and concern that their bosses would not see unemployment and its effects on health as legitimate issues for health workers to tackle. This last concern may be particularly important, and some health workers trying to persuade unit and district managers to adopt strategies for responding to unemployment and health have met considerable resistance. They are not opposed to individual health workers being trained in unemployment and health but do not see that there is any need for them to take any action, or receive any training, themselves. But many, including the Unemployment and Health Study Group, would argue that individuals will find it very difficult to be effective unless they are encouraged from above and are working within a coordinated strategy.

What can doctors do about unemployment and health?

- Recognize problems in their patients caused by unemployment
- Know their patients' occupational histories
- Refer their patients for advice on benefits
- Know of national and local initiatives to help the unemployed and so be able to refer patients
- Work locally to make people aware of the health consequences of unemployment and so help to reduce the stigma of unemployment
- Consider organizing employment schemes either alone or with the Manpower Services Commission

---

Another factor that is likely to be important is the attitude of some health professionals towards the unemployed. After my articles were published in the *British Medical Journal* some doctors wrote to the journal saying that they thought that many of the unemployed could get jobs if they wanted and were choosing to be unemployed.[3] The implication was that they were lazy scroungers. Some correspondents went further and suggested that the unemployed should not reproduce and that the young should be conscripted.[4, 5] These stigmatizing and victim-blaming attitudes are common among the general population, and may be widespread among health professionals—nobody wrote to take issue with our correspondents. They are exactly the attitudes that help to make unemployment so painful, and if many health professionals do think this way then it is not surprising that the health response has been so feeble.

Before a strategy can be developed for responding to unemployment and health, the authorities—from the top down—must recognize that unemployment does lead to health problems and does increase the workload of health agencies. This the government has now done. Norman Fowler, Secretary of State for Social Services, wrote to Michael Meacher MP, his opposition counterpart, on 1 July 1985 to say: 'I would not question that unemployment may well have negative effects on health, though by no means in all cases. I agree too that people who are unemployed need to be helped by those with whom they come into contact, including the social services, to overcome the negative effects of unemployment.' Mr Fowler also made the point in his letter that his department was monitoring research on the relation between unemployment and health and using it to formulate policy. But advice from the health departments to regional and district authorities on how to respond to the health implications of unemployment is conspicuous by its absence. Nor does the health of the unemployed feature much—if at all—in government discussions on creating jobs or reforming the social security system.

The first responsibility of the government should be to take account of the impact on the health of the unemployed of its own policies, and to this end the Unemployment and Health Study Group advocated an interdepartmental committee with exactly this brief.[4] Secondly, the government should be monitoring the impact of unemployment on health and encouraging research. The evidence that I have is that such research has been more discouraged than encouraged. Thirdly, the health departments should be advising health authorities on how best to respond to unemployment, and they should be taking regional unemployment into account when resources are distributed. Fourthly, they should be pushing for the training of all health workers to include something on unemployment and health.

At the moment, as far as I can see, the government is not doing any of these things. Yet the government has shown—with its response to drug addiction among the young—that once a long-neglected issue becomes a matter of national concern something (albeit of doubtful effectiveness) can be done quickly.

Health authorities need to draw up strategies for dealing with unemployment and health, and the report published by Strathclyde Regional Authority could serve as a useful blueprint.[6] The strategy should summarize for staff some of the convincing evidence that unemployment harms health and then state the authority's commitment to reducing the harm. One of the main jobs of an authority will be to monitor the effects of unemployment in its area and then perhaps to target responses at those most in need. Regional authorities will also need to consider taking unemployment levels into account when distributing resources.

The authorities should have a policy of sharing the employment they have to offer as much as possible and should also consider how they can create work either on their own initiative or in co-operation with the Manpower Services Commission. Information for staff and the unemployed on the huge range of facilities available to the unemployed should be the next component of the policy, and the authority should appoint somebody to assemble a directory and then make it available to all its staff. This should be combined with training key staff in what can be done for the unemployed and with seconding some staff to local community initiatives. Authorities should also make arrangements to provide counselling to unemployed people who want it. This could be achieved both by encouraging individuals within the authority and by perhaps establishing a special unit.

Action tends to come about only when individuals are made responsible for coordinating and stimulating initiatives, and each authority might appoint such a person. One of his or her main jobs might be to liaise with other health authorities and with local authorities to avoid duplication of effort.

A survey of all the regional health authorities, all district health authorities, the health boards of Wales, Scotland, and Northern Ireland and the family practitioner committees of England and Wales showed that many are beginning to do something, although none has a published plan to match that of Strathclyde Regional Council.[7] Harris and Smith did not send a questionnaire but rather a list of seven activities that the authorities might be undertaking. Respondents were invited either to respond to these suggestions or to respond in any way they wanted.

The overall response rate was 76 per cent (251/331), comprising a 72 per cent response from the district health authorities and health boards (158/219) and a 90 per cent response from the family practitioner committees (88/98). Most of the regional health authorities did not consider it their job to produce a plan to respond to unemployment, but three were doing something—two working with the Manpower Services Commission, and one allocating resources on a formula that took some account of unemployment.

Nor have many family practitioner committees taken much action on unemployment, which is not surprising as the committees have only recently been given powers that might allow them to take any action—and most do not yet know what they can do and do not anyway have any money to do it. One responded: 'We have only just learned to walk and have no shoes.' Despite this, four committees are monitoring local unemployment, one is relaying information on unemployment and health to staff, four are taking unemployment into account when allocating resources, ten are participating in job creation, seven are giving advice on facilities and benefits, five are liaising with local authorities, and five are targetting responses at those most in need (Table 13.1). This seems not a bad start for organizations without shoes.

District health authorities and health boards are doing much more (Table 13.1). Almost two-thirds of the respondents were doing something, and almost a quarter were taking three or more of the suggested steps. (Fig 13.1 shows which authorities were doing something and how much they were doing.) Authorities with high unemployment were significantly more likely to be responding than authorities with lower unemployment, but many with high unemployment were not taking any action. Several respondents said that they were not taking any action because they had low unemployment rates in their district. In October 1986, however, only three local authorities in Britain had unemployment rates under 7 per

TABLE 13.1. Response of health authorities to the health problems of unemployment

Step	No	1	2	3	4a	4b/5	6	7
Health authority								
Regional health authorities	9	0	0	0	2	5	0	1
District health authorities and health boards	158	33	15	20	65	55	13	23
Family practitioner committees	??	4	1	4	11	7	5	7

1   = monitoring unemployment and its effects locally
2   = relaying this information to staff
3   = taking unemployment into account when allocating resources
4a   = creating jobs and work
4b/5 = training staff on facilities for the unemployed
6   = liaising with local authorities
7   = targeting responses at those most in need

Note: The questionnaire by mistake had two number 4s. As most respondents considered the second 4 (4b) and 5 together we have lumped them together in our analysis.

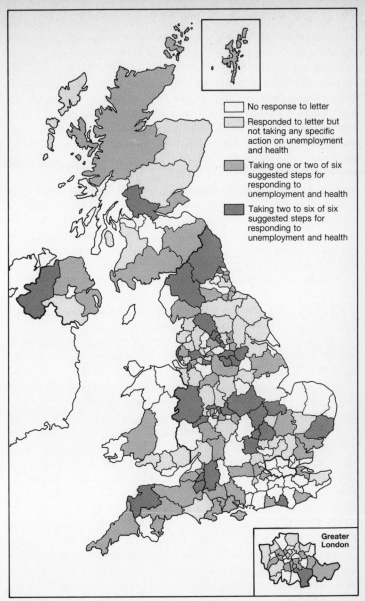

No response to letter

Responded to letter but not taking any specific action on unemployment and health

Taking one or two of six suggested steps for responding to unemployment and health

Taking two to six of six suggested steps for responding to unemployment and health

Greater London

FIG. 13.1 Response of district health authorities and health boards to the health problems of unemployment.[7]

cent—and even that would have been thought of as a high rate just a few years ago. This sounds like a poor excuse for inaction.

The medical Royal Colleges and organizations such as the British Medical Association, the Royal College of Nursing, and the Health Visitors Association all have an important part to play in encouraging research and discussion on unemployment and health, gathering together information, and disseminating it to their members and to the public. At the beginning of the book I asked whether we would eventually see a report from one of the Royal Colleges on unemployment and health. If we ever do it may well come from the Royal College of Physicians of Edinburgh. It has undergone what the *Scotsman* has called a quiet revolution, and its new president—cardiologist Professor Michael Oliver—is quoted as believing that 'at the heart of current health concerns are those related to poverty in the midst of affluence'.[8] He wants the College to take action on poverty, and in doing so he is taking the College back to its roots. The guidebook to the College's headquarters points out that in 1861 'the 21 original fellows were concerned not only with the advancement of medicine as a reputable science but also with ways of alleviating the miseries of the poor and needy'.

Two national bodies that perhaps have particular responsibility to do something about unemployment and health are the Health Education Authority and the Scottish Health Education Group. The unemployed tend to be scattered and alone but could be reached by health education initiatives that provided information on how unemployment might harm health and on what could be done to minimize the harm. The information could tell people where they could get advice on benefits, training, and other initiatives and could give ideas on healthy diets on low incomes and on strategies for coping. The Greater Glasgow Health Board health education department has already produced a pack on unemployment and health that could serve as a model.[9]

Individual doctors and health workers, particularly those working in general practice, can do a lot to help the unemployed and their families (see box on p. 185). Firstly, they can be aware of the harm associated with unemployment and can make certain that they know their patients' occupational history. The long-term unemployed are those most at risk, but also to be watched closely are the middle aged with heavy commitments, those deepest in poverty, those who are repeatedly in and out of jobs, and those who have been obliged to accept early retirement.[10, 11] The second responsibility of doctors and their staff is to make sure that patients are getting all the benefits to which they are entitled. The general practitioner need not do this himself but should be able to point his patient towards somebody who can help.

Thirdly, health workers should be able to tell their patients about local and national initiatives to help the unemployed. (We obviously cannot publish a list of all the initiatives in Britain, but the box on p. 192 gives some useful national addresses.) Fourthly, they should try to make their local communities aware of how unemployment can harm health and should take the lead in reducing the stigma of unemployment. Fifthly, health workers as employers and organizers should consider what they might be able to do to create work for unemployed people.

No doctor has ever been taught any of this at medical school, and many will consider that tasks such as these should not be part of a doctor's job. But, as Brandon, a professor of psychiatry, has written in a leading article in the *British Medical Journal*: 'Depression associated with the problems of parenthood, unemployment [or] poverty . . . is often relieved more by practical interventions than by formal psychotherapy or drugs.'[12] Furthermore, as the Royal College of General Practitioners has emphasized, management skills are becoming increasingly important in general practice,[13] and the general practitioner need not do all this work with the unemployed him or herself. Responding to this problem will be a challenge to the 'modern general practitioner', and it is one that few have yet taken on.

Finally, much more research needs to be done on unemployment and health, and perhaps now as health authorities and workers wake up to the immense implications of unemployment for health, grant-giving bodies will be more willing to back research. If they are going to do so what research is needed?

The *Lancet* has argued boldly that no more research is needed into unemployment and health: 'If government excuses inaction by claiming that it awaits the outcome of research, academics should not connive.'[14] It seems extraordinary to argue those researching into unemployment and health are somehow conniving with government inaction, and the fallacy in the argument is surely the implication

National sources of help and information for the unemployed and people caring for them

Manpower Services Commission
Moorfoot
Sheffield S1 4PQ
(There is a national network of
  Job Centres)

National Association of Citizens'
Advice Bureaux
115 Pentoville Road
London N1 9LZ
(There is a national network of
  Citizens' Advice Bureaux)

TUC Centres for the Unemployed
Trades Union Congress
Congress House
Great Russell Street
London WC1B 3LS
(Directory of centres available, price £3)

Unemployment Unit
9 Poland Street
London W1V 3DG

Unemployment Alliance
26 Bedford Square
London WC1B 3HU

Unemployment and Health Study
  Group
5 Lyndon Drive
Liverpool L18 6HP

British Unemployment Resources
  Network
Birmingham settlement
318 Summer Lane
Birmingham B19 3RL

Centre for Employment Initiatives
140A Gloucester Mansions
London WC2H 8PA

Church Action with the Unemployed
318 St Paul's Road
London N1

Child Poverty Action Group
1 Macklin Street
London WC2B 5NH
[Produces a poster on benefits
  (price 75p including postage) and two
  handbooks—*National Welfare Benefits
  Handbook* and *Rights Guide to Non
  Means Tested Social Security Benefits*
  (both £4 including postage)]

Strathclyde Regional Council
*Unemployment—Implications for
  Regional Services.*
Available from:
Chief Executives Department
Strathclyde House
20 India Street
Glasgow G2 4PF

Black, D., Laughlin, S., eds
*Unemployment and Health: Resources,
  Information, Action, Discussion*
For information and copies contact
  authors:
Health Education Department
Greater Glasgow Health Board
225 Bath Street
Glasgow

South Sefton Health Authority
*Guide to the MSC Community
  Programme*
Available from:
Health Services Management Unit
Department of Social Administration
University of Manchester
Manchester M13 9PL

that the government would take action if academics stopped their research. Watkins has argued that 'little is to be gained by studies designed simply to ask whether unemployment is bad for people'.[15] This seems a fair proposal, but have researchers ever undertaken such naïve studies? Surely the aims of most studies, although rarely achieved, are to try to quantify the harm done to health by unemployment, to determine whether the unemployment or the harm comes first, and to determine whether it is the unemployment itself—rather than its usual accompaniments—that causes the damage.

Thus I would argue that there is still room for basic studies that explore topics such as the effect of unemployment on women and families. Much needs to be done, too, to look at whether unemployment itself causes a deterioration in health; Watkins argues for a study along the lines of Stafford *et al.*,[16] but one that looks at physical rather than psychological health. (This study was important because it proved—in a way that has never been done for physical health—that unemployment causes psychological ill health.)

But I do accept—as Watkins argues—that one of the main thrusts of research should now be to look at how unemployment harms health—the 'intervening variables'. Work like this has been done and more is in progress, but its importance is that it might allow a more intelligent response to alleviating the harmful effects. In the same vein, the second main thrust should be intervention studies that explore the best ways of helping the unemployed.

References

1. Unemployment and Health Study Group. *Unemployment, health and social policy.* Leeds: Nuffield Centre for Health Service Studies, 1984.

2. Popay, J., Dhooge, Y., Shipman, C. *Unemployment and health: what role for health and social services?* London: Health Education Council, 1986.

3. Anonymous. Occupationless health. *Br. Med. J.* 1985; **291**: 1427.

4. Christopher, C. Occupationless health. *Br. Med. J.* 1985: **291**: 1427.

5. Monro, J.K. Occupationless health. *Br. Med. J.* 1985: **291**: 1427-8.

6. Anonymous. *Unemployment—implications for regional services.* Glasgow: Strathclyde Regional Council, 1985.

7. Harris, C., Smith, R. What are health authorities doing about unemployment and health? *Br. Med. J.* 1987; **294**: 1076-9.

8. Dinwoodie, R. President prescribes remedy for college of physicians ills. *Scotsman* 1986 January 17: 11.

9. Black, D., Laughlin, S., eds. *Unemployment and health: resources, information, action, discussion.* Glasgow: Greater Glasgow Health Board Health Education Department, 1985.

10. Warr, P. Twelve questions about unemployment and health. In: Roberts, R., Finnegan, R., Gallie, D., eds. *New approaches to economic life.* Manchester: Manchester University Press, 1985.

11. Daniel, W.W. *A national survey of the unemployed.* London: Political and Economic Planning Institute, 1974.

12. Brandon, S. Management of depression in general practice. *Br. Med. J.* 1986; **292**: 287-9.

13. Royal College of General Practitioners. *Quality in general practice.* London: RCGP, 1985.

14. Anonymous. Unemployment and health. *Lancet* 1984; **ii**: 1018-9.

15. Watkins, S.J. Recession and health—the policy implications. In: Westcott, G., Svensson, P.G., Zollner, H.F.K., eds. *Health policy implications of unemployment.* Copenhagen: World Health Organization Regional Office for Europe, 1985.

16. Stafford, E.M., Jackson, P.R., Banks, M.H. Employment, work involvement, and mental health in less qualified young people. *J. Occup. Psychol.* 1980; **53**: 291-304.

Index